George Baker began teaching Physical Culture before the last war, after a short and successful career in various sports – including Australian Rules Football, Amateur Wrestling, swimming, running and cricket. He is an expert on Hatha Yoga and has trained in Ballroom Dancing in order to study its value in health and fitness. Mr Baker has been teaching Physical Culture for nearly thirty years and benefits from his own extensive training programme.

Keep Healthy :
Stay Younger

GEORGE H. BAKER

Australia's leading physical fitness expert

SPHERE BOOKS LIMITED
30/32 Gray's Inn Road, London WC1X 8JL

First published in Great Britain by Pelham Books Ltd 1970
Copyright © George H. Baker 1970
Published by Sphere Books 1975

TRADE
MARK

Set in Monotype Baskerville

Printed in Great Britain by
Hazell Watson & Viney Ltd
Aylesbury, Bucks

ISBN 0 7221 1419 2

KEEP HEALTHY : STAY YOUNGER

INTRODUCTION

In writing this book I feel that some outline should be kept in view of the scope of the readers who may be interested. It has been written therefore to cover a variety of aspects of healthful living so that an overall pattern of staying healthy and maintaining youthfulness is presented. Technical depth has been avoided as I feel that the average reader does not want a text book but rather a guide to better health and being younger.

I propose therefore to cover a range of subjects suitable to all age groups and objectives. The chapter on nutrition can be of use to everybody wanting radiant health and the chapter on mental approach and psychological attitudes can help the person who has problems regarding the doing of exercise. Yoga for the beginner will be most beneficial to all who wish relaxation and better health and could be done by everybody even when doing the other exercise routines. A chapter on dancing and recreational exercise is included as this activity has an excellent value for physical and mental health.

I feel that in this highly technological age with its stresses and strains, its polluted air, denatured foods, status symbolism and the race to keep up with competition, some positive effort must be made to combat the wear and tear and ageing stresses besetting us. With mental disorders on the increase, also alcoholism, plus the effects of drug and poison induced diseases, lung cancers, coronaries and the damaging effects of smoking, is it not high time we took stock of the effects of such highly civilized living on the body?

Some deep thought and positive action are necessary,

some constructive moves for better health, some counter-prevention of the modern killer—tension. We need to use our bodies the way Nature intended we should and endeavour to nourish it that natural health way with food as Nature grows it, unadulterated, unrefined.

This book is written with the objective of showing how to exercise, how to eat, how to relax and live a healthful life and be younger.

CHAPTER ONE

Why Bother?

In this age of tremendous scientific expansion with the emphasis on man's most priceless possession—his magnificent brain and the fact that he survives by the use of it, one often hears the question asked—why bother using our bodies, the muscles, why exercise? At first thought and indeed to many people with further thought, this question may seem a good one. If we are surviving, keeping alive longer (though not necessarily more healthfully) making a good living, having a good time enjoying life by using our brains, indeed we might ask why bother to exercise our bodies. We do not have to use our muscles to do things, go places; we have automobiles, trains, planes and other transport, we have automation in the home, industry and generally labour-saving devices that our grandparents had never known.

One might point out further that the time that we would have to use up for exercise could be used for pleasure and recreational pursuits. After all is not the objective of fast automation to make more money, give us more free time and generally make life easier; so why use this extra time in exercise, sport and exertion; why bother, it seems so unnecessary, so much like 'hard work' and for what? Why not leave all this to the athlete, the youth with ambition for sporting fame and to the boy or man with the desire for big muscles and strength and to exercise cranks, the show-offs, fanatics and the people who need strength and muscular fitness in their jobs perhaps.

To the person who thinks along these lines and who may ask these questions one may say in reply that if they want no better health than that which they now have through living that sort of life then don't bother. If that person is so made that they can live in superb health by living that sort of life then that person is indeed lucky, a very rare animal and would be a source of wonderment for physiologists and all scientists concerned with the animal body. We have all heard people state that they live in good health, have no diseases and feel fine and that they never exercise and are never concerned with the food they eat or with any practices to improve health, or fitness. Indeed they are only too ready to tell us this and boast that they are fit and do not need exercise or crank diets. It is a fact, of course, that quite a few are naturally blessed with a very fine constitution and do at first glance appear to be as they boast they are, but it is also a fact that these same people do not carry this health very far into or past middle age. Even the best of constitutions will show some signs of neglect and begin to lose efficiency.

These same people quite often also tend to forget to mention that their appearance is not their natural one and that they did have two 'colds' and mild 'flu' last winter and that a few times they had a bit of indigestion and occasional headaches and tiredness that could not be explained by late nights. They might also say that everybody has these little things wrong with them at some time or other. It could come as quite a surprise to them that there are people who do *not* get these little things wrong with them. One also hears the very well worn statement they are 'a little bit fat' because its their nature, their parents were fat and above all this they really do not eat much at all. When it is pointed out to them that their idea of eating 'not much at all' is still well above their calorific requirements, the alibi—equally as well-worn— is that they have to keep their strength up, could not possibly eat less, would starve and so on. Some, a little more honest with themselves, and with their fellow men and women, will admit that they are lazy and love their food, while others will not admit these characteristics but nevertheless know it in their own conscience that they are in that latter category. As for exercising, why bother, it makes them tired, interferes with their pleasure and takes valuable time. They do not realize that it takes much less time than sickness does and costs far less. We always find time, in fact, we are forced to find time for sickness when sickness hits us.

A little time spent in exercising and generally practising healthful living will prove that it is worth the bother. The rewards for the effort involved are plenty. The increased stamina for one thing gives more time before fatigue catches up, and so we still have the time available for pleasure and recreation plus more vitality for the use of it. Further, the exercising period, far from being spent in reluctant boredom can be spent in pleasant company, in bright surroundings and can be combined with recreational activities if in the form of social games, such as tennis, golf, hiking, swimming and many other combination social exercise activities. We meet people with a similar outlook and objectives and this can be stimulating mentally as well as providing perhaps a spur to our efforts and to push us along by competition when we begin to falter, or become bored, or when laziness tends to override our good intentions.

The increased enjoyment of life that will be experienced will be a reward for bothering and our relationship with people around us improves with the improvement in health with the radiance and magnetism with which a really fit body shines. We all have felt the depression, slight or pronounced, that can be felt in the presence of a personality complaining of aches and pains and the boredom of being told of a person's illnesses and feelings of fatigue, the dullness and lack of sparkle that seems to be around such people. How much nicer and more stimulating to be in the presence of health and vitality and indeed to be the centre of it ourselves and radiate the magnetism and personality that makes one's company sought after and enjoyed.

Superb fitness and tireless health enables a person to enjoy the company and the activities of people of all ages, to join in their fun and games and be one of them. Age is no bar if fitness is ours. How tragic to be old at 50, to be too worn out with tension, wrong food and slothful living, to enjoy much more of life. Is it not worth some little bother to avoid this, do we not all of us want more out of life, do we not all of us, some secretly perhaps, admit that we would like to have the vitality and freedom from aches and pains that really is our birthright? We are sick because we violate the wonderful laws of nature that she made to keep us brimful of pep and health. We are not meant to be old at 60 or thereabouts, youthful vitality and vigour can be maintained much longer than that. We wear our bodies out with disuse, abuse and dissipation, over-indulgence in food and drink—we rust away.

Tension, mental stress, worry, fear, anxiety and apprehension are today our great enemy. Rise in blood pressure, ulcers, insomnia, the inability to relax, are an accompaniment of this tension anxiety state so prevalent. The increased percentage of cholesterol in the blood in many cases is due partly to tension and anxiety. The excessive stimulation via the nervous system of increased adrenaline into the blood stream whips us up for fight or flight, neither of which we do in the amounts necessary to use up our hormonic whip. The result is that we remain, in some cases, constantly in a state of fear and tension. Add to this the habit of reaching for a cigarette 'to calm us down' and we have a further kick to the blood pressure, not to mention the poisoning effect on the system generally, the irritation of lung tissues and in fact all other tissue and cell which is directly in line of contact of the smoke.

The question which emerges here is why bother with exercise, what can that do regarding all this tension and anxiety and stress? A trial will soon convince that it can indeed do plenty and in many cases very quickly and markedly. Physical tiredness is quite relaxing in contrast to mental fatigue which is not conducive to sleeping. Exercise could be worth the bother for this alone, but we have the further benefits of keeping the blood vessels young and more elastic, the drop in blood cholesterol, the increased efficiency of the heart and lungs, youthfulness both in appearance and in keeping actively young and bright in our outlook. Our ability to play the games of life, is not really a matter of age, it is more a matter of the preservation of the capacity of the animal body to repair itself, recuperate vitality with rest, 'recharge our batteries'. This we can do only if our body is maintained at top tuning, we cannot afford to be clogged with food, stale with our own waste products, flabby from not using our muscles, lacking digestive keenness because we are not truly hungry, mentally fatigued and testy because we cannot sleep soundly. Correct exercise and faithful application of principles of health can produce this condition of 'top tuning' which can enable the body to give us the bounding vitality, optimism, freedom from little aches and pains, the sound sleep and happiness and enjoyment that we should have.

Fatigue is brought about by many factors, healthful and unhealthful. Healthful fatigue is the only desirable one, of course, and for this one must use the muscles and body to the stage of relaxation. There is no more relaxing tiredness than that produced by the healthful activity of games or systematic exercise; there is no truer hunger than that produced by a hard session of exercise, be it a workout in a gymnasium, a hike through bush country or a recreational game of some sort.

True hunger today in a modern civilized community is rather a rare phenomenon, it tends to be replaced more by the false appetite, the eating by the clock, the eating at social gatherings, business dinners and luncheons. The person who has not experienced a true hunger from really natural physical need for food will be pleasantly surprised at the difference in actual taste of food, the increased enjoyment and digestive efficiency. The food being quite definitely needed physiologically rather than psychologically will be more readily digested and assimilated.

Too many meals today in our highly civilized life are eaten because it is time to eat, we knock off for lunch, we have unnecessary mid-morning and mid-afternoon snacks and a 'cuppa'. There is rarely any true physiological requirement at this time, it is habit, false appetite and quite often a seeking of diversion from the boredom and monotony of our task. Eating, like sex, is a most powerful primitive instinctive compulsion. These two very primitive instincts are along with the instinct for self preservation, the most powerful driving force in our existence and quite frequently are closely inter-related. An example of this close psychological interchange or crossing of instincts is the fact that sex starvation drives many people to turn to eating, and eating in large amounts, compulsively. One instinct is starved, the other is satiated; but all too often, far too extensively. Thus we have one of the basic causes of over-eating and in a particular age group, teenage and middle age frequently.

14

The regular practice of sport or some systematic exercise regimen can do wonders to help overcome the harm of such over-eating and quite often also is a definite sublimation of the sex drive surplus. The hunger for food is more natural while the energy for sex drive is to a certain extent sublimated and thus we may get a certain balance or evening out of these instincts of basic needs and desires. The mental state of tension and frustration tends to lessen and we are more likely to approach that state of peace of mind, happiness and contentment that we do all so much want and seek.

To the young man indulging in some competitive sport will also come the added satisfying of the instinct to compete and win, a further balancing out of our instinctive drives. It is said that there is less delinquency and crime amongst the athletic man indulging in sport, with an objective of fame and honour than amongst the idle youth on the street corner. Some pride in the body's appearance and ability is present in all of us. The youth with the inferiority complex is faced with the poor alternative of outlandish dress perhaps to focus attention on himself, or some cult or activity to draw attention away from the poor appearance of his undeveloped body. The lust for power can sometimes be seen in the driving of a fast car or motor cycle, the appearance of being 'big' with a cigarette so held and smoked ostentatiously. How much more admired and respected is the clean cut athlete, healthy and fit, vital and virile, confident and calm? How much greater value to the community is such a person? How much less overcrowding of hospitals, surgeries and clinics would there be if we had more of such types? The economy of a nation with a predominance of fit people would be raised greatly. Examinations of recruits for military service provides us with a shocking revelation of just how unfit we are. Surely it is worth the bother, in fact it should be incumbent upon us to make the effort for these reasons and our own personal benefit.

It would come as quite a shock to most people to learn just how much the upheaval and domestic break-ups that occur can be traced back to the unhealthful conditions of people, the effect of alcohol on the family with a heavily drinking father, the irritability of a chain smoking executive type father, tense, nervy and jumpy, or the same condition in a mother, bored, affluent, with little to do, becoming obese and seeking unhealthful reducing techniques.

A hobby of healthy gymnasium activity or games is well and truly worth the bother of cultivation. The value to people in such cases is inestimable and has the further unselfish value of making others, namely the family, happier and with a greater assurance of security and domestic peace. In the rat race of today's anxious striving to get ahead (or even to stay where we are and not be submerged) the winners and survivors are the mentally equipped and physically fit. These two attributes are more closely bound today than ever before. Mental disorders are on the increase, we are not yet able to cope with the intense mental anxiety that is so hand in hand with the strivings for security and improvement of our lot. We must be physically fit and tough to be really mentally fit. The old saying *mens sana in corpore sano* was never more applicable and never more necessary. We owe it to ourselves, our family, our community, and our country to make the effort and bother to get ourselves as fit as we can in our civilized conditions. Air pollution, denatured food, soft living are today part of our daily environment and we can do something about this by practising some form of healthful activity, in clean air where it can be found, finding out where we can obtain 'natural food', compost grown and free from pesticides, artificial growth with artificial fertilizer.

We will be well rewarded, it is worth the effort and the value for time involved is a much greater return than any money we might make by impairing our health. Many a rich man is too old and worn out at 50 through making his fortune, to enjoy the fruits of his efforts, his money cannot buy the health and youthful vitality with which he started out. How much better to be just merely comfortably secure and reasonably well off but be able to enjoy life fully, and able to indulge in everything without fatigue, side effects or pain.

Whether or not we believe that exercise and healthful living can give us longer life or whether we believe that heridity determines exclusively the number of our days on earth, the fact remains that healthful living with attention to exercise and diet and healthful thinking does give us more enjoyment of the days we do have and prolongs our youthful feeling, and defers the final slowing up as we near our end. Nevertheless plenty of people do die of diseases which can be prevented and so it could be said that they would have lived longer if they had taken some measures to keep really fit and avoid sickness and degeneration due to neglect of the elementary laws of nature regarding care of their bodies.

Even if a person does not take any serious steps at health and fitness promotion, better mental and physical health can be his or hers if they at least avoid the dissipation that so much has become part of modern living. Excessive drinking and smoking, high living and tension do not have to be a necessary condition of living in a modern civilized society, but they nevertheless seem to be accepted as such. Perhaps we are afraid not to conform, how many people have their first alcoholic drink merely to be 'in it', their first cigarette to feel and look adult as they think. Lack of courage to face this without being too conformist is probably a factor in the beginning for many a person's first harmful venture. Recent evidence of the harm of smoking points to a very wide range of troubles that plague the heavy smoker. The lung cancer chances would appear to be the most emphasized but the evidence shows that heavy smokers are much more prone to cancers and disorders of most other organs and tissues of the body. Heart disease for one is high on the list and a smoker stands a much greater chance of a coronary than a non-smoker. The list is long indeed but more of this in later chapters.

One may ask how this can be affected by exercise and diet. The answer is that exercise can maintain the tone and elasticity of the small blood vessels, the lungs and the heart; it increases the elimination of poisons from the body and decreases the cholesterol level, ensures sounder sleep and improves digestion and assimilation of food. Even if one does not care much about being really fit, is it not still worth the bother to do something to offset to some degree the harmful effects of a dissipating type of existence or as one gentleman so aptly said 'to enable him to do better, the things he should not do at all'. How much better—if one cares to indulge in peculiar rationalizing—to be fitter to stand up to dissipation and fitter to do the things we should not do at all.

CHAPTER TWO

The Value
of Exercise

When considering and discussing the value of exercise to the body, we should, and in fact we must, realize the different values to different people, age groups, and sex, and the different value of different exercise. What would be of considerable value to a youth interested in muscular development would not automatically be of the same value to a middle-aged person. Exercise for muscle building—which is largely weight resistant type of exercise —is not as beneficial to the heart and lungs as would be that of a cardio-vascular-pulmonary type, of which distance running and swimming are good examples. It is this latter type of exercise which proves to be the more healthful to middle age—partaken of course with due thought to the condition of the person. Coronary trouble being the high relative risk condition from middle age onwards, it seems quite desirable, and essential in fact, that the type of exercise most helpful in prevention of these prevalent coronary risks should be the exercise that most works the heart, lungs and blood vessels in a steady but not exhausting manner. It is a proven fact in the physiology of exercise that the heart benefits most from a steady, prolonged and mildly enduring session, rather than a violent burst occasionally.

Trotting, jogging, steady easy running for a distance of 2 - 3 miles daily, or even merely 3 - 4 times per week, has a wonderful tonic value to the body generally, and the toning effect on the arteries, arterioles and capillaries, of the constant, steady dilation, contraction and pulsation, is of tremendous 'prevention' value in avoiding heart attacks, 'strokes' and circulatory disorders, with their side effects. Even regular walking, taken for its value in healthful frame of mind and not merely to get from point A to point B, can be of great help. In fact, in the early stages of a person's course of action, it may be desirable and advisable to begin with it, and then graduate to steady trotting.

Even when running is being regularly indulged in, walking should still be done everywhere possible. Too many people today use the automobile to travel 100 yards or less to the corner shop for a small shopping item. Statistics can show us that the occupations with less coronary trouble are those in which walking or movement is involved, and conversely those with high figures of coronary trouble are the inactive, sedentary ones. These figures of course are subject to considerable variation with the influence of cigarette smoking, and the locality, whether it be city or country air.

The value of exercise to the youth during teenage maturing is of mental and physical nature. The whole future of his manhood is largely moulded in these developing years, and the physical foundation is necessary for the health and constitutional strength he builds up, and the mental confidence that comes with it as a more than fringe benefit. The instinctive urge in developing youth to excel, win, prove itself, is too often seen in the louts who attack in numbers an innocent person, instead of on the field of sport or in a gymnasium. How rarely does one hear of a Judo expert, boxing champion, or wrestler, attacking anybody? They do not have to prove to themselves, or to anyone else, what they are capable of doing, or how manly they are. The value of the psychological make-up of a person, of building a body that can be admired for its appearance and the sporting feats of which it may be capable, cannot be fully estimated. One can perhaps judge fairly well if one thinks of the number of class sportsmen, and realizes just how few of these people are not pleasant personalities and desirable company.

It must be realized that muscular development is a prime factor that influences many young men to begin a physical training programme, and so the exercise suitable for these objectives must be used. If the person is concerned with training for any specific sport, the building of muscle is still of importance because it can be, I think, true that strength is always an asset, added to the skill of an athlete. In fact, no doubt would exist in any person's mind that, two athletes being of equal skill and experience, the stronger one will win. The muscle building routine of course must not, if the person is concerned with a 'speed' sport, be such as to cause loss of speed. The emphasis in these cases should be on the greatest possible increase of strength for the least possible gain in actual bulk. Some gain will naturally take place, but far too many body builders place too much value on bulk, and train for this purpose with high food value diets and additives, to the detriment of skill and endurance. Of course, if the person is not a competing athlete or sportsman, and is training merely for body shape and bulk, or winning 'Mr.' contests, then the whole objective is centred on and around exercise for this purpose. The value of such exercise is quite specific for this objective.

Body building and development

The comment is frequently heard when a man of exceptional muscular development is observed, with a muscle size and shape that has obviously been built by a systematic training programme, 'Who wants all that muscle—what's the use of it—what's the value?'; 'What happens when he knocks off training?', etc. One also hears quite frequently from girls and older women also that they do not like 'all those horrible muscles', 'it looks repulsive', and so on. Such men are quite frequently accused of being mirror athletes, narcissistic, and even homosexual. With such comments and opinions, it could be quite natural to ask what is the value of such an exercise routine. It must be understood, of course, that such comments are not a majority expressed opinion, but are, particularly from youths and poorly built men, quite obviously envy and a repression of secret wishes to be the same. In fact, very few men, if offered the gift of 'instant muscular perfection', would refuse it. Laziness, and the lack of drive to get down to real hard work, are the reasons, in some cases, why most youths and men do not possess well-developed bodies. Heredity, of course, determines just how good our potential, but nevertheless considerable change of shape can be wrought in the body by the continuous training of an exercise programme. There is no short cut. Hard work and determination are the essential elements in the building of muscle bulk and shape. It can take years to reach the stage of being a champion.

The value of an exercise régime or course designed and set out for the purpose of developing the muscular system is firstly in the improved strength and power that becomes obvious. It is not true—as some people have thought—that muscle built by such method is not really strong. It *is* strong—no muscle built by hard work is merely big. It is a very well-known fact, of course, that two men can have a muscle measurement exactly the same size, and in all respects be the same build and weight, and yet one can be quite clearly stronger in actual strength tests—leaving out skill. The influences of the nervous impulses and the leverage insertion of the muscle are largely responsible for this, and it could be said perhaps that one person has actual better quality muscle fibre.

The value of strength alone is something that one needs to experience to appreciate. In any walk of life, or sport or activity, real strength is no load to carry—unlike fat, which is much more than a load, being in fact quite harmful. Insurance companies can supply figures to prove this. The value of handsome shape is appreciable when we see a person with such—the straighter posture, the masculine taper, the graceful movement, etc. The psychological value and ego boost are greater than most people realize, and of considerable benefit to the building of confidence and morale. Even though an exercise course for muscle building is usually mapped out for hard weight resistant work, and does not usually include stamina or endurance work to any large degree, a 'side effect' of such a programme is noticed in increased stamina, and certainly increased fitness and health.

The value of hard weight lifting routines for the middle aged is perhaps debatable. Since the principle requirements and results sought after by middle age or older men are largely health and reducing and the prolongation of life, and the avoidance of disorders, it is probable, and in fact preferable, that exercise programmes be for their category less violent or heavy, and more of the steady heart, lung and blood vessel toning type. A very well developed upper arm is of very little value to a man in the prevention of a heart attack, but a slim abdomen and sufficiently conditioned heart and lung functioning with elastic arterial response, is a far more preferable and valuable asset. The value of exercise then for this person lies more in the nature of the exercise than in just doing any exercise, although to a degree any exercise is better than none. Exercise tolerance varies considerably from person to person; we are not the same when it comes to speed, strength and power, and value of exercise done is naturally greater or less for each of us, but still nevertheless valuable to our physiology.

The value of exercise as a relaxant is not fully realized and appreciated. A person very tired from work and mental occupation does not feel like doing exercise. Nervous fatigue is all too common, and it is quite a difficult job to convince such a person, tired from such mental tension, that exercise will relieve the tiredness and not make one more tired. Complete relaxation and healthful sleep of sound quality, and not merely restless quantity, are not possible in a body which is tense and nervy. Use of the muscular system wisely will definitely reduce tension and lessen the fatigue. The adrenalin secreted by the adrenal glands is not used up for the purpose for which it was secreted—namely the requirements of the muscular system in emergencies of physical effort more strenuous than normal. The influence of fear, with its possible follow up of flight or fight in primitive conditions for physical survival, is to produce this extra secreting of adrenalin to enable the quicker mobilization of blood sugar from the liver, to raise blood pressure, increase arterial circulation to the muscles whilst decreasing it to the intestine, the dilation of coronary artery circulation, and generally preparing the body for greater efficiency of physical effort in flight or fight. If this keyed up state is not resolved or relieved by the physical effort for which it was created, then the tension is retained and with tiring effect. It is an all too unfortunate fact that modern civilized conditions of life are constantly creating tension and subconscious fears, and unless we do something about it we are wearing our bodies out with this nervous tension. It is by means of good vigorous exercise that we can release and relieve this tense state, and relax. The effect of tension and anxiety on digestion is only too well known, and so relaxation becomes even more essential for the best digestion and assimilation of nutriment.

The value of exercise, particularly taken in clean, cold air, on the complexion and skin generally, is quite evident by the healthful rosy colour that comes with it. There is no better beauty treatment than a healthy blood stream flowing through a skin toned by clean, cool air, with vigorous circulation and happy relaxed frame of mind. The complexion of women in Northern European climates is well known for its clearness and beautiful colour. The so-called drying out and wrinkling of skins exposed to air is not really so traceable to the air, but more likely caused by the constant washing with hot water and soap, and perhaps the polluted city air and dietetic lack of skin foods, and excess of harmful foods.

The physiological effects of exercise are quite noticeable and measurable as regards the actual changes in the blood during exercise and following it. The increase in the white corpuscles has the effect of increasing the body resistance in the fight against disease and infection. Certain corpuscles are increased in number, the reason and purpose of which is not too clearly understood, but of which it is most unlikely to be anything but beneficial. The increase in numbers of red corpuscles and the oxygen carrying capacity is well known, and the benefits and value of this physiological fact are quite obvious and well realized. It is not within the scope of this book to elaborate with detail on the physiology of exercise—there are many very good text books on this subject and branch of physical training science. It will be sufficient to note here that the effects of exercise on the biochemistry in the body are quite profound, and are largely subordinated to the needs of the muscular system and the fitness of the body to accomplish tasks and endure physical effort, and which improves with regular systematic training. The condition of the trained athlete is so superior to the untrained, unfit man that no further proof should be needed to convince any person of the value of exercise for better health and fitness.

Many people will argue that they do not need the fitness of the trained athlete. This is so—they do not perhaps require the peak fitness of the highly trained sportsman; in fact the athlete himself does not maintain such peak, but endeavours to be at this peak for a particular event, such as a boxing championship. However, there is a point below which it is courting actual ill-health to allow the fitness to decline. In view of this, is it not a desirable safeguard against poor health and sickness to at least maintain a degree of fitness to keep one free from aches and pains, fatigue, depression, and generally feeling out of sorts?

To attain and retain this level of health and fitness, exercise is essential, even if not to the rigorous schedule of athletic or sporting requirements. The value of the mental make-up that comes with the feeling of confidence in being able to resist infections, stand up to tiring work, and still have energy and vitality to play and enjoy life, is appreciated mostly when one looses this degree of health and fitness. The retaining of youthful energy to a ripe old age is something we would all love to do, and the morale boost to the person ageing in years, but not in looks and feeling, is considerable. What better uplift to a woman in middle age to be assured that she looks no older than 35, or less.

Retaining youthfulness in the human body is not so very different to maintaining efficiency in a machine. The human body is itself the most wonderful machine of all, but like all machinery will rust if not used, and will wear out with abuse and disuse. Also excessive strain and wear and tear on any particular part over a period of years can produce symptoms of pain and decrease efficiency. It is desirable to exercise and use all parts of the body, and regularly so. Some exercise daily is preferable with light days, and perhaps one or two work-outs per week of rather vigorous effort. The value of a good puff daily is inestimable, and we should aim at this. Like all purchases, value for money is a desirable objective, so is value for exercise taken—we get back what we put into it; the loafers have the least fitness, get least value for money or effort spent. On the other hand those most amply repaid with the best results are those who have put something into it. For these people the results and value are a bargain, and the attainment of something more precious than money— perfect health. Many a millionaire would trade a fortune for a new stomach, new heart, new kidneys, or set of glands. What good is money without the health to enjoy what money can buy?

The value of sport and games for persons other than those in the fierce professionalism of big time, or the dedicated of top amateur games—Empire, Olympic, European, etc.—is still basically a desire to excel, even though not perhaps with the killer instinct, or win at all costs attitude. Although this mental attitude, and perhaps the reason for playing, may be social also, the exercise value is still there, perhaps not so great, because most social players of tennis, golf, bowls and the like do not go into training for their sport. Whether we train rigorously for sport as a youth, or are merely once a week players without serious training, we are getting exercise and reaping value and rewards that we otherwise would not have. The hiker who walks through the bush and hills merely for the love of the bush and air, is getting one of the healthiest benefits of exercise. Walking is our most natural means of getting somewhere, but we do all too little of it unfortunately. As an exercise it ranks very high; it can be done for longer periods than most other exercise or sport, and provides a steady and lengthy exercise for heart, lungs and muscles, without violent strain.

The value of exercise from walking is found to be one of the most beneficial for post-coronary heart attack, and is a very excellent beginning for an exercise regime designed to build heart health. The lead up to gentle jogging is ideal, and prepares the heart for something a little more vigorous, such as climbing stairs and squat exercises, and the capacity to participate in dancing and social activities.

One value perhaps not fully realized or appreciated regarding exercise is the psychological one that we can do things if we have to in emergencies. We have confidence in our capacity, because we know that the exercises that we have been doing have been tough enough to enable us to do most household jobs and work. We tackle a heavy concreting job, a heavy digging job, and suchlike, with the knowledge and confidence that we should not 'do our back' or have to spend hours in hot baths, or even bed for the next few days. Many a 'back trouble' has started because the person has not been a regular exerciser, and has tackled a lifting job or attempted some difficult manoeuvre that the body was not in condition to handle. The value to our ego and confidence in knowing we can do anything in reason that crops up is a most appreciated one.

Exercise benefits that are not too well known, in fact hardly realized by most people, are those benefits that may be called fringe benefits. In this category we can include the eyes. The eye muscles themselves are used in different and healthful way in a game of tennis, or any sport requiring eye co-ordination and focus, and this is of great value in relieving the strain and tension of office work and reading, television, cinema, etc. The value to our feet of romping around barefooted on lawns and sandy beaches is much underrated. The relief to congested metatarsal heads and arches is considerable, and what woman does not feel relief and benefit from such a pastime. In actual fact, the value to health of such effects of exercise on the eyes and the feet is really not a fringe benfit, but just merely an unrealized benefit of unrecognized value. Do we not all know how tired we feel all over when our 'feet are killing us', how our back will ache if we walk with a limp or in such a way as to ease our 'barking dogs'. Likewise the headache that can accompany eye strain and fatigue. The relief of headache from tired eyes, that can be had by doing a few simple neck exercises with breathing, has to be experienced to be appreciated. If to this routine of neck exercise we add actual exercise of the muscles that move the eyeball itself, and the muscle of accommodation, then we can very largely eliminate future troubles and strain, and many a person has discontinued the wearing of glasses from such eye culture.

The value of exercise to the skin should be most obvious to people; most of us have noted the healthy glow after an afternoon in the fresh air playing golf, tennis, etc., or after indulging in a solid training session. The increased circulation to the skin cleans it, nourishes it, and even oils it.

Our body, our muscular system, was made to be used. Despite the fact that modern life has dulled our appetites for doing just this, nevertheless deep down amongst our primitive instincts we really can relish movement and activity. After all, movement is life and life is movement. To enjoy life is to enjoy movement, and to enjoy life the most we must have movement. When modern living prevents natural moving, then we must needs substitute specific exercise to give us this movement. Our bodies love it; we must bring our minds to love it also, as the value to both is inestimable, and we must accept the realization that it is necessary and must be done if we are to have the health and fitness that is possible for us.

There are many of what could be called 'hidden benefits' and values of regular exercise indulgence. These are the benefits to the small blood vessels, the ligaments in various parts of the body, and various benefits physiologically that do not show up so obviously at the time, but which are apparent in later life. We find that we retain better circulation, have more flexible and pain free movements in parts of the body where poor blood flow and poor flexibility are so common in many people in later life. Better circulation to areas of the skin where age begins to show can defer the wrinkling we dread. Wrinkling plus fatigued appearance is very aged looking, and the value here of Yoga exercises is tremendous.

We do not really know perhaps the full value that we obtain from a regular exercise programme. We certainly can see much of the beneficial changes in a person who takes up exercise after years of slothful dissipation and wrong living, but much of the benefit and value is inside also, and becomes apparent in emergencies of accidents, stresses and strains of civilized living.

When one appreciates the differences in young children deprived of ample play facilities from those with unlimited opportunities for play and games, one can realize just how important exercise is for the growing child. How much brighter and alert is the youngster who can give full play to the natural instinctive desires of the young to play, wrestle, and generally do the things that children will naturally do. All young animals will play, wrestle, run, jump, climb and use their growing bodies in every way. Kittens, puppies, and domestic animals generally are observed readily and no better example is available. Watching children at play, one constantly hears adults express the admiration of the energy displayed. The value of play, exercise and natural movement to the growing youngster needs no elaboration, as it is so obvious.

We would not have to stretch the imagination too far to calculate the beneficial effects to us if we could still do these things in middle age, and even old age. How youthful it would keep our bodies and equally so our minds and mental outlook. The value of a youthful outlook, with a backing of experience and the wisdom of age, is something that would make life so much more enjoyable.

CHAPTER THREE

Food and
Healthful Eating

The time was not so far past when fitness was thought to be merely a matter of hard physical training, early nights, sexual abstinence and plain food. Today, any athlete who regarded this as all that was necessary for peak fitness would find his own peak so far below that of more scientifically trained men that he would be left wondering and wanting.

The science of nutrition, food values and healthful eating has progressed at a rapid rate over the last thirty years or so and no programme of physical fitness or training would be complete or comprehensive enough to ensure results in the hurly-burly of today's struggle to live or excel in sport. The 'plain food' is no longer plain food. It does not contain today what it contained in the past and on the other hand it does contain additives, chemicals and preservatives which are not healthful even though they be in small quantities that do not show any immediate harmful effects. Add to this the devitalization of our common foods like bread and cereals and we have a very common cause of one of the great deficiencies of our modern diet—lack of the Vitamin B Complex. The further loss of this vitamin together with Vitamin C in wrong cooking produces an even greater struggle for the body to retain glowing health and fitness. There are still plenty of people who take no special care of what they eat, and who maintain a reasonable degree of fitness and even some athletes who win championships. A high degree of skill and vigorous training physically can carry these athletes through, blessed as they mostly are, with a very strong constitutional inheritance, but stamina and endurance events can sometimes show out dietetic deficiencies.

The terrific resilience and recuperative power of youth and early manhood and womanhood is a further asset in enabling people to 'get away' with wrong eating. However, the day of reckoning eventually comes and the athletic life of such poor eaters is usually much shorter than that of a person whose diet is studied and scientific; the lapses of form more frequent, and the injury proneness much greater, the recovery time much longer, the weight problems more difficult. Overeating is probably the great killer of form and health for the athlete and the ordinary person. A famous authority a few years back once said that people eat twice as much as they need and that they live on only half of what they eat, the medical profession and the undertakers live on the other half. I am inclined to agree with this.

The question arises now as to just what is the proper diet for anybody, athlete or otherwise. The old saying of 'one man's meat is another man's poison' comes to mind and though I would say that there is a certain amount of truth in this I would say also that there is health and benefit for all from a certain standard of eating. We must, of course, exclude allergy here as this is specific and personal. The old argument of meat eating versus vegetarianism crops up and never really gets settled. There are champions who live almost on meat, and others who are complete vegetarians. The question also is debated as to whether added vitamin or mineral or both have any value or are necessary, likewise added protein compounds. Regarding this latter one could say that this is definitely overdone. Stuffing the body with extra protein merely throws greater strain on the liver and kidneys. Many a bodybuilder shows symptoms of mild kidney trouble and liver complaints with complications such as haemorrhoids. We must not lose sight of the limitations of the bio-chemistry of the body. We can assimilate only a certain amount of protein concentrate and this is much smaller than most people think. Merely eating large amounts of high protein foods in concentrated powder form or tablets in addition to a high meat and egg diet does not auto-matically ensure that the muscle will get the benefit. A great deal of chemistry takes place before this stage and the body's capabilities cannot be strained too far, too often in the quest for muscle. Likewise certain vitamins can be quite toxic if taken in excess, namely Vitamins A and D.

These latter are fat soluble and this of course could be a contributing factor to toxic effects because of liver involve-ment and possibly congestion. Water soluble vitamins appear to be less harmful in excessive amounts. In fact, Vitamin C appears to be very highly tolerated in large amounts up to as high as hundreds of milligrams daily. Excess is passed out in the urine with no more discomfort if any, than a rather acidic urine. Vitamin B complex on the other hand can produce some very strong manifesta-tions of excess by unpleasant skin rashes, 'nerves', etc., diarrhoea, digestive upsets, but these symptoms may pos-sibly be due more to an imbalance between the B family as much as a total excess.

An excess of Vitamin B_1 for example can produce symptoms of B_2 deficiency in some cases. The difference between synthetic single Vitamin B concentrates and food extracts of natural vitamins of the B family is quite significant. Molasses, yeast, wheatgerm, etc., are all high Vitamin B foods but more important are rich in more than one of the Vitamin Bs and in the balance and proportion that nature produces them. Yeast has the further benefit of containing a high proportion of the essential amino acids, the building stones for protein synthesis. These latter foods are much more beneficial than the dosage of single synthetic Vitamin B particularly as they contain usually rich mineral concentrates as the iron, calcium and potassium in molasses. This latter has been found to be of immense health value for intestinal shortcomings, bowel and digestive, and greatly lessens the discomfort and inflammation of haemorrhoids.

It has been stated that it is not necessary to add vitamin concentrates to a diet which is generally well balanced with meat, eggs or fish, fresh vegetables and fruit, wholegrain breads and milk, butter and cheese. This may have been so in the days when food was not processed, refined, preservatized with chemicals, artificially coloured and generally robbed of its mineral and vitamin content by these refinements. We do need to make some addition to our diet of vitamin concentrates to make good this loss. It is preferable, in fact, one may say necessary, that the added vitamin and mineral be in the form of food extracts such as molasses, wheatgerm, yeast, rather than synthetic single vitamins.

Vitamins are destroyed in various ways by heat, oxidation, exposure to light, and drugs, smoking, chemicals such as pesticides, etc. As our foods are now rather heavily loaded with such poisonous chemicals, does it not seem necessary to add to our diet the extra vitamins so needed. If further losses occur with improper cooking it is no wonder that the average plain food diet is definitely deficient. Boiling with plenty of water, added salt and soda all bring about the destruction of vitamins and the loss of minerals, more specifically the B group and Vitamin C. The eating of a daily raw vegetable salad and plenty of fresh fruit together with bread and cereals that are 100%

pure wholegrain becomes an essential if health is to be maintained.

Vitamin A

The importance of vitamins in the diet can be fully appreciated when we see the results of their absence. Vitamin A deficiency shows up with weakened resistance of mucous membrane of the respiratory tract, also the gastro-intestinal tract, to diseases. Its value in the prevention of night blindness is well proven. Vitamin A is essential for healthful growth in the young and is a skin beautifier. Exposure to air can cause unstable reactions but it is not affected by heat. It is also suspected that cold storage causes some deterioration. It is found in rich quantities in fish oils and vegetables such as parsley, spinach and carrots. Cheese, egg yolk and butter are also good sources.

Vitamin B Group

Although deficiencies of any single B Vitamin can occur, most Vitamin B deficiencies are probably multiple as the vitamins of this group are mostly in combination in certain foods. Lack of this essential group can produce a host of ailments such as poor appetite, lack of vitality and vigour, skin troubles, headaches and nervous debility, fatigue, neuritis, eye trouble and heart disease. It is essential for growth and digestion and assimilation of food, healthful peristalsis of the intenstine and bowel. Probably the most notable of symptoms of deficiency is the disorder and malfunctioning of the nervous system.

The Vitamin B family are water soluble and as such cannot be very readily stored and so need to be replaced daily for health. There are some eighteen or so members of this family, over half of which can be made chemically. Between them they are vitally concerned in a great diversity of functions, amongst which the most important could be listed prevention of fatigue, keeping the skin healthy, assuring the nervous system, maintenance of a healthy digestive tract, prevention of premature old age and grey hair, healthy eyes and hair. Each one appears to have specific functions and the deficiency of any one member can produce specific symptoms, but quite often multiple symptoms manifest themselves as deficiencies are more likely to be in more than one of the B family. Functions of some of the lesser known members are not too well understood but the glands, hair growth, and healthy liver functions are influenced by para-aminobenzoic acid, inositol, and folic acid. The importance and function of Vitamin B1 in the prevention of fatigue is well proven, likewise Vitamin B2 for the skin and eyes, B6 for healthful nervous relaxation.

Vitamin B foods fortunately are found together in natural foods and it is far more beneficial to obtain them from this source than with tablets or isolated shot in the dark, hit-or-miss balance, or guess work. Some foods contain many of the B Vitamins in rich amounts, others only a few, but the overall consumption of a wide variety of vitamin B rich foods would ensure a balanced supply and prevent deficiencies. Unfortunately the foods which are richest in the Vitamin B family are not eaten daily by most people and in many cases not at all. A further contribution to B Vitamin deficiencies is made by the refinement of our grain products such as the use of white flour for bread, the polishing of rice and generally the refinement that takes place in the preparation of these foods. To avoid Vitamin B family deficiency all refined cereals and breads should be avoided, and the following foods liberally eaten and made a permanent part of daily diet, not necessarily all of them in any one day but as many as can be used. Molasses—probably the richest source of pantothenic acid and inositol—should be a daily addition, yeast —a very rich source in a large number of Vitamin Bs, wheatgerm, soya beans—also very valuable protein— vegetable oils, particularly corn oil and wheat germ oil which are rich in B6. Raw foods such as parsley, watercress, spinach are rich in folic acid and as this vitamin is very quickly destroyed by heat, it is essential that these types of foods—intensely green leafed—be eaten raw and daily.

Fortifying white bread and refined cereals is in no way a natural replacement and balancing up and is very little better if any than the original refined product. To obtain a balanced supply of Vitamin Bs and ensure against deficiency the daily diet must include helpings of these rich foods. The amounts needed vary considerably with different people. Highly strung, nervous individuals would need perhaps more than a calmer more sedate and peaceful type. The amount of exercise taken also influences the requirements and the hard training athlete needs much more than the less active person. Men perhaps need more than women and also perhaps the ratio of Vitamin B family requirement varies with persons. Children need ample of the growth promotive B Vitamin, notably Vitamin B2. Even where there may be lack of exact knowledge of the precise functions, the food contents and the requirements, we cannot go very wrong if we follow the plan of eating as nature provides and eat some raw green foods daily, molasses, vegetable oil, yeast, and consume only unrefined cereals and 100% wholemeal breads, nuts, soya beans and certain seeds such as sunflower and sesame.

A very valuable source of many of the B Vitamins is cultured milk such as yoghourt and buttermilk, etc. These contain bacteria which thrive in the intestinal tract and have the ability to synthesize some of the Vitamin Bs especially folic acid and biotin which are very influential in the maintenance of good health. A further added benefit and a very considerable one is the fact that these rich Vitamin B foods contain valuable minerals, molasses for instance being very rich in iron, copper, calcium and magnesium and potassium. There is no guesswork with mother nature and Vitamin B deficiency can be avoided by careful attention to avoiding the wrong foods and eating the valuable natural raw ones.

Of all the Vitamin B rich foods, dried brewer's yeast is the most valuable because of its high content of so many of the B Vitamins, and the fact that it contains all of the family in some degree. Add to this the high content of minerals and amino acids and we have a complete Vitamin B and protein rich food plus an abundance of essential minerals. It can be taken in tablet form if unpalatable to some tastes, but in powder form can be stirred into fruit juice, milk, vegetable juice and soups as a daily insurance against deficiency.

Vitamin C

Vitamin C or ascorbic acid is a daily essential vitamin in the preservation of resistance to infections, preventing allergies and poisoning or toxic effects of foreign substances which may have entered the bloodstream. It is helpful in preventing fatigue, and the appearance of old age, and the consequent preservation of looks and youthful vigour. It is an essential building stone in formation of connective tissue, and maintaining strength and elasticity of ligaments and cartilage. The walls of the blood vessels are strengthened and together with Vitamin P is a valuable preventative of 'strokes' and haemorrhage. Deficiency results in slow healing of wounds, and adequate amounts greatly speed up the healing of cuts, wounds, broken bones, ulcers and injuries generally. Early symptoms of deficiencies are bleeding gums and easily bruised tissues and slow healing. Vitamin C is found in all fresh fruits and vegetables, the richest sources being citrus fruits, black-currant juice, tomatoes, cabbage, rose hips, and acerosa cherry. It is not stored in the body and needs to be supplied daily for radiant health. The amount varies but excesses are more tolerated than deficiencies so it is best to have an adequate amount of all fresh fruits and vegetables. It is needed in greater quantities in illnesses such as fevers, infections, arthritis and rheumatic complaints, allergies and post surgery and also when drugs are used extensively. It has been found also that cigarette smoking greatly increases the need for Vitamin C intake. Large helpings of fresh raw fruit, salad vegetables and lightly or waterless cooked vegetables should be a daily essential in the diet as this vitamin is destroyed by cooking and oxidation.

Vitamin D

Vitamin D is largely concerned with the formation of sound bone structure, and teeth as it is necessary for the efficient metabolism of calcium. It is found in fish oils and fats but it is doubtful if the quantities are adequate. We obtain it by sunbathing as the sun's rays act on the oil in our skins and synthesizes it but as so much of the oil is washed off by the use of soaps and excessive hot water we can quite easily be under supplied. The consumption how-ever, of concentrated sources of this vitamin is not to be advised as it is quite toxic in excessive daily amounts and adequate amount would be obtained from a reasonable supply of fat in the diet plus exposure of the body to sunlight, particularly avoiding the use of soaps and hot water to excessive degree on the days of exposure.

Vitamin E

Vitamin E has been found to be an essential for reproduction and growth and healthful pituitary gland function. It has been used widely in the treatment of heart weaknesses and appears to enhance and strengthen the heart beat. It greatly heightens the ability of the body to utilize oxygen with consequent improvement of muscle functioning and has been used with success although doubted by some authorities, for athletes indulging in endurance sports. It is especially beneficial in circulatory shortcomings and with attention to mineral requirements of the body, proved very valuable in the prevention of chilblains.

Vitamin K

Vitamin K is necessary for healthful and speedy blood clotting and is found in green leaves. It is apparently not destroyed by heat but being soluble in fats it cannot be readily assimilated in the intestine without healthy production of bile salts, nor readily assimilated with consumption of paraphin oil.

Vitamin P

Vitamin P has, like Vitamin K, a role connected with haemorrhage. However, its function is concerned with the blood vessels and the strength of same. It prevents porous conditions and fragility of the smaller blood vessels and lessens the danger of rupture and bleeding and possible strokes. It is said to greatly help in the reduction of high blood pressure. The richest source is lemon peel, but it is found in citrus fruits generally and certain types of green peppers. Rutin has been used with considerable benefit for high blood pressure.

The vitamin family of essentials are not completely known and possibly many are yet to be discovered which will be found to be essential for perfect health. The vitamins unknown as yet will no doubt be found in our food—natural and as it grows, and the consumption of raw natural food will ensure us an adequate supply of the known and unknown. In fact some are now known to be essential for animal life and will no doubt be essential for humans. Balance appears to be very important in the intake of vitamins and it might be prudent to assume that the taking of concentrated single vitamins in tablet form is not in natural harmony with nature and it would be a far less margin for error and imbalance to get our vitamins in the form of raw natural foods and extracts such as molasses, yeast, wheatgerm, etc.

Although man is omnivorous with his eating habits, it does not follow that eating many varied foods in any one meal is not harmful. Most animals eat only one food at a time and many only one food all their lives. There is no doubt that many of man's digestive deficiencies and ailments are brought about by the complex mixtures of so-called foods that are shovelled into the stomach in one sitting. Add to this the smothering on the food of excessive salt, pepper, mustards, sauces and condiments generally it is no wonder the stomach together with the liver is man's most outraged organ. To add insult to injury, meals are almost invariably washed down with tea, coffee and topped off with a cigarette, all of which have harmful effects on the ease and rapidity of digestion. So many meals today are also taken in haste under tension and very insufficiently masticated.

Fasting

Fasting is unknown to the vast majority and to miss a meal would not only be a hardship unendurable to most but would create a mild panic because of the symptoms that may follow, mental and physical. The truth of the matter is that a fast would be the greatest tonic to the insides of modern people and the much needed rest to the digestive system most appreciated. Fasting enables the body to have undivided attention to the task of cleaning the body, repairing and rejuvenating, catching up with elimination of waste products and burning up of excess fat. A one day per week fast as been advocated by many health authorities, and longer fasts of 3, 7 or 10 days once or twice a year have worked such wonders in the restoration of health that we would be well repaid to use a little will-power and have regular fasts. Simple meals, thoroughly chewed, are far preferable than exciting exotic dishes, spiced and got up to tickle the palate and incite appetite. True hunger requires none of this tempting but will be well content with a simple natural single food. The unfortunate circumstance of modern man's food habits is that in an affluent society true hunger is virtually unknown and is replaced by false appetite. This latter is so governed by the clock that it could be also termed habit appetite. The regulation of our daily life is of course such as to render it difficult to eat any other way but by the clock. It could be overcome to a certain extent by not eating unless we are really in need and to be sure of this one needs to have done some hard exercise or eaten very little for a considerable time. As the weight of most modern people is on the fat side it would seem that this regular eating is not what it has always been thought—necessary. We must create a physiological need for food, not merely be tempted to eat because it is time and the food looks delicious. If the food is concentrated regarding calories value our problem is of course much more difficult and we more than ever need the hard session of exercise.

The excessive consumption of bread, biscuits, cereals, etc., washed down with milk is all too common a breakfast and unfortunately not the most healthful. Very few people in fact really need a heavy starch meal so early—they have not had time to get hungry and would be far better off on a light fruit meal. Milk itself particularly pasteurized is not the wonder food for adult human beings. It is very mucous forming and adds greatly to the catarrhal conditions so prevalent and many a child's tonsils and adenoids condition can be cleared by avoiding pasteurized, creamy milk. The calcium value is not readily assimilated because of the changes brought about by pasteurization.

One of the greatest menaces of our modern diet undoubtedly is refined white sugar and products containing it. No greater robber of calcium and valuable mineral exists and the dental condition of the average person is ample evidence of the damage of this harmful chemical. Its effect on the digestive tract also is quite known and the fermentation and acid forming qualities of this denatured product are quite harmful to the maintenance of health. White sugar contains no vitamins, minerals or protein and should be avoided strictly and appreciated for what it is— a source of unwanted calories and a deficient and harmful chemical substitute for food. The sweet taste is acquired just as the taste for salty, spiced foods and any person accustomed to a natural diet of raw, unsalted, unsweetened foods finds sweetened food unpalatable. Common table salt, sodium chloride, is also quite unnecessary and in fact harmful when used sprinkled on food or cooked into food. This is not to say that we do not need salt—we do—but we are meant by nature to obtain it in natural combination in raw foods, not cooked out and then replaced in inorganic sprinkling on our plates. The so-called requirements through sweat loss have been proven to be almost a myth. A properly balanced diet of plenty of raw, fresh fruit and vegetables with no excesses is capable of supplying all the salt needs. The adjustment with sweat loss is readily made.

Excessive salt can produce kidney irritation and other troubles such as water retention and a circulatory disorder and is known to be quite harmful with high blood pressure and heart disorders.

One of the greatest sins of modern day eating habits is most surely that of overeating. Nothing is easier to do, no sin has more alibis, no habit other than drug addiction harder to break. The causes are complex and include mental and physical, emotional and biochemical. Anxiety, stress, unhappiness, frustration, both sexual and in the business world, repression, loneliness, misfortune and many other side effects—all contribute to over indulgence at the meal table. Sometimes deficiencies of vital bio-chemical elements or compounds in our diet cause an unrealized craving and we eat more in an effort to get sufficient of the required nutriment. An example of this is the craving of pregnant women on some occasions, also the excessive craving for sweets with a protein deficiency.

We must choose our food more wisely, selected from only the wholesome abundance of Nature, unspoiled, unrefined, unsalted, unsugared, not artificially coloured or preservatized. Further, we must not cook it wrongly but should eat more of it raw as in salads and fresh fruits. We must chew it thoroughly and we must eat in calmness and peaceful atmosphere and not when tired or when not really hungry. Most of us do not really need the traditional three square meals per day but it is a sorry fact that this idea still prevails and most people eat not only three square meals per day but add a couple or more extra between times. If the three square meals were spread out over 4 or 5 hours and were not too heavy we would be better off, but it is all too common today for the civilized stomach to not be empty completely, and rested, before another meal is heaped into it. Is it any wonder that the over-worked stomach has to throw in the sponge every so often and demand a rest?

Adequate amounts of Vitamin B are needed for good digestion and healthy strong peristalsis of the intestines. Molasses *has* specific effects on the intestinal functioning and is very helpful in constipation and haemorrhoids. Honey is a very valuable adjunct to the diet and should be used in all sweetening in preference to white sugar. Its properties include digestive aid, intestinal purifier and liver benefits. It is antiseptic and a bowel aid and invaluable with cider vinegar or lemon juice in throat and chest troubles. The virtues of cider vinegar have been mentioned in many pamphlets and booklets. The mineral content and richness of available oxygen make it excellent for blood and intestinal disorders.

We are what we eat. If what we eat is pure and wholesome we can expect to be the same. If on the other hand what we eat is lacking in vital necessities we will be the same and health will be lacking in that sparkle and radiance which Mother Nature meant us to possess. Even the exceptional muscular strength possessed by some men is not a safeguard against sickness and disease. Examples of this are quite readily found amongst the apparently superbly fit athletes, footballers weightlifters, boxers, wrestlers, swimmers and others. The relatively high rate of colds and influenza would suggest that in spite of the excellent physical fitness of these men, something must be wrong for them to get illnesses such as these common ailments. Exposure to the cold and wet with footballers cannot be the basic cause, for indoor athletes get colds and 'flu and other common disorders. The basic cause would logically appear to be in the food they eat. Large appetites brought about by hard training very often are the undoing of their fitness. Too often overeating is all too easily indulged in and in this fact we have a very common root for sickness, particularly as the diet is largely the wrong one. Some sports and training methods have not kept up with the modern research and nutritional science developments; old ideas die very hard, and even today many athletes still adhere to the belief that steak must be the main part of the diet, and many still have a large steak preceding an event.

The over indulgence in starchy foods also is a mistake most frequently made and as the bread, cereals, biscuits and such foods are largely made from refined white flour we have a deficiency for a start. The disinclination to have much fruit and salad vegetable in the winter diet with the subsequent overbalancing with hot cooked dishes, stews and the like further adds to the deficiencies, particularly in the very vitamin we need in large quantities to help prevent winter ills—Vitamin C.

The sicknesses afflicting athletes at Olympic and inter-country games is most likely due to the different food and the fact that many athletes have their national dietetic habits induces many of them to bring much of their own food with them. Visiting teams quite often loose fitness to some degree and frequently have more injuries than the home team. Coaches in some sports have kept ahead with nutritional developments. Researches in the physiology of exercise is still a fairly recent study, and much more could be learnt yet to add to the proficiency of our athletes through better nutrition, and much more training and experiment done. In some sports the coaches and trainers are often, in fact nearly always, ex-champions with their old ideas of fitness and all too little educated or trained in the more scientific and up to date ideas regarding diet. They lack the knowledge of food values and dietetic health facts.

The value of diet in the healing of injuries is not fully appreciated, likewise the value in preventing same. The role of Vitamin C is very significant in the strengthening of connective tissue such as tendon and ligament. It further has the property of aiding in the reduction of rheumatic inflammation and this is more common than realized in athletes. Vitamin E is also thought to play an important role in the muscle tone mainly because of its circulatory benefits and its ability to help the body utilize oxygen more economically and particularly the heart muscle. Some authorities doubt this and have discontinued adding Natural Vitamin E to the diet, but my personal experience has produced only benefits and greater performance, and I have seen much benefit to elderly people and heart patients.

A popular idea with many athletes is the one that milk is essential. Milk has many excellent properties but it also has many factors against it. It is very mucous forming, constipating, and the fat content not easily digested and inducive to cholesterol formation. When pasteurized it is not easily digested generally, and the calcium content largely unabsorbed and wasted, the Vitamin C content very small and it has practically no iron. I cannot agree that it is a natural food for man, most particularly adult man. No other animal naturally goes on drinking milk after weaning, but man not only does so, but drinks that of another animal. Some compromise has been made in this direction by removing the fat and consuming the skim mostly in powder form with consequent higher relative protein ratio. The basis of most high protein muscle powders is this skim milk combined with soya bean powder, yeast powder, egg powder and perhaps wheat germ. The consumption of such potent combinations should be limited however because the body's biochemical ability to handle such protein concentration is not unlimited, and over enthusiastic indulgence can quite often produce symptoms of liver congestion and disorders of the bowel. In fact, the consumption of all concentrates, including

Vitamin and protein, mineral, etc., must be done with an eye for symptoms of excesses likely to cause disorder to liver, stomach and bowel. The blood pressure should be checked, the urine analysed and tested occasionally and the fatigue susceptibility looked into. Heavy consumption of meat is not necessary. The soya bean has a higher protein percentage than most meats plus the added benefit and healthful properties of lecithin and high percentage of alkalizing minerals and vitamins. Eggs should be taken in moderation even by the body builder. High cholesterol content makes it a danger food for the middle aged or inactive man or woman and quite a deal of liver congestion and conjunctivitus are the result of consuming too many eggs, particularly fried and with meats.

One of the habits that causes us much trouble is the one of improper or insufficient mastication. This is brought about partly by the fact that a large proportion of our foodstuffs is wrongly prepared, overcooked and mashy, and does not induce chewing, in fact, renders it hardly necessary at all in some cases. A greater proportion of raw food in our diet would give us the need for more chewing but even with this inclusion many people would continue with old habits. One must be made aware of the need to chew and make a conscious effort to chew more thoroughly.

A further contribution or more correctly a major reason for insufficient mastication is the nervous, tense state of many people and the hurried eating that is so universally common today. Too often eating a meal is done in too noisy an atmosphere, too many people and too much attention being paid to conversation. Witness the undivided attention that an animal such as a dog or a cat gives to a meal and how important it is to them. We tend to regard a meal as a social event or a business discussion or deal and the natural habit of hard chewing and taking time over a meal is something seldom seen. Further, a large proportion of people are really rarely truly hungry but suffer more from a feeling of emptiness or 'pangy' feeling which is not true hunger but largely the acidic remains or fermentation of a badly digested previous meal. The instinct is to fill the stomach and fill it quickly, no time to waste in chewing.

True hunger is rarely felt in the stomach itself and never is felt as a pain or even pang. Contractions of the stomach take place when it is emptying but surely Mother Nature does not intend hunger to be painful. False appetite and time clock eating are so common today that the stomach does seem to protest if it is not filled regularly regardless of whether or not the body actually needs food. The bulging waist lines and overweight bodies so prevalent today would tend to lend weight to the fact that eating too regularly, hungry or not, is really only another form of overeating.

Digestive shortcomings probably are the most common and frequent ailments prevailing today. A large proportion of these shortcomings fall short of actually producing symptoms of indigestion, but merely are such that while no pain is actually manifest the food is not completely digested and passes on without the maximum benefit that should be assimilated from it. Added to this the factor of Vitamin B complex deficiency so necessary for digestive efficiency and we have the ideal set up for digestive troubles, small at first, but sooner or later with symptoms—and pain. The difficulty of digestion of some foods is another factor that should be considered. In many cases one meal is not fully digested and cleared before another one is tossed in on top of it. Is it no wonder the overworked, outraged stomach is forced to rebel and protest. Many stomachs in fact, are in a constant chronic state of catarrh and mildly inflamed. This state is usually, if not almost always accompanied by some form of liver congestion or disfunction, mild or noticeable. The eventual result is seen after years of abuse to these organs—gastric and duodenal ulcers, gall stones, gall bladder disease.

As a guide to healthful eating in the selection of foods the following list should be consulted and used. I do not suggest that it should be followed to the letter religiously but the more strictly one does the better the nutrition of the body and the digestive efficiency.

The following foods *should be avoided* always: —

1. Refined sugar (white) and products containing it or made from it such as jams, jellies and sweets, etc., sugared fruit juices, syrup drinks, etc. and chocolate.

2. All white flour products, white bread, and cereals and grains, refined denatured, white rice, etc., pearled barley.

3. Salted foods and all condiments, sauces, pickles, mustard and such.

4. Saturated fats and hydrogenated oils, coffee, tea, cocoa and alcohol, tobacco.

5. All roast meats, fried foods, smoked and salted meats and preservatized meats such as sausages and the like. corned meats, hot dogs and such like.

6. Excessive dairy products and eggs. Dried fruits containing sulphur dioxide. Chickens fed with drug foods and hormones.

7. All foods containing preservatives, artificial colouring and chemicals, additives, vitamin enriched or with stay fresh properties.

8. Overcooked vegetables, stale or stored foods and foods grown in excessive pesticide conditions.

The following foods *should be eaten* but in moderation, according to the calorie requirements and weight control: —

1. Wholemeal bread and whole grain cereals, unpolished rice, etc.

2. Honey, molasses, black treacle and raw sugar (sparingly).

3. Polyunsaturated margarines, unsalted for preference, and vegetable oils such as Safflower, Soya, Maize and the like.

4. Skim milk, soya bean milk, yoghourt, buttermilk.

5. All nuts, and seeds such as sunflower and sesame. Health sweets made with honey, nuts and lecithin, etc. All meats grilled for preference. Fish steamed or boiled.

The following *should be eaten daily* in plentiful quantity: —

Fresh fruit—1–2 lbs. minimum. Salad vegetables— other vegetables steamed or waterless cooked (potatoes in jacket). Soya beans and products from Soya bean.

Best drinks—preferably diluted with *distilled* water— cider vinegar, unsugared and unheated fruit juices without added preservatives. Herbal teas, dandelion coffee, and cereal coffees. Vegetable extract drinks.

The selection of foods for daily requirements should be made with consideration for both nutritious value and health, and calorie needs. Restrictive selection of the concentrated starch foods such as breads and cereals should apply, while unlimited—within reason—selection of fresh fruits and salad vegetables may be made.

Endeavour to space meals at least five hours apart, but this can be lengthened or occasionally shortened between some meals having regard to speed of digestion of the previous meal. For instance, after an all fruit meal, the next meal could be as close as two–three hours. In any case never eat unless really hungry—missing a meal is an excellent tonic. Endeavour to be hungry, earn your meal physiologically, take time to chew thoroughly and endeavour to be relaxed and in a peaceful atmosphere.

CHAPTER FOUR

Psychological Approach and Mental Attitude

Mind and body are bound together in their functioning for our health. No true peak fitness is really possible unless the harmonious interfunctioning of mind and body is present. The effect of mental stress, sadness and unhappiness, frustration and worry all have deep reaching effects on our bodily chemistry and healthful functioning. The poor digestion from mental stress, the lack of desire for food in unhappy love and loss of loved ones is all too well known to us but never fully appreciated. The ever present fatigue and weariness of the unhappy person, the bored person and the under privileged is around us daily.

This same psychological effect is carried into the athletic world. The top athlete needs to be free of worry and mental problems if he is to perform at his top. Domestic peace and security are prerequisites for good health, sex security and compatibility are necessary, freedom from mental boredom and happiness in one's job are all vitally necessary for completely healthful functioning of the body. Financial worry and hardship all have their effect on our energy and stamina. Although this mental fatigue makes us feel disinclined to exercise, the fact remains that exercise is most necessary here and the person invariably feels better after it.

One of the most difficult obstacles or barriers that we encounter in the pursuit of health is the laziness and disinclination to exert ourselves. We are so surrounded with inducements and facilities for doing things the easy way that people who take the stairs in preference to elevators are quite often called fitness cranks. The automobile, the bus, the railway, all take us to places all too often that could be walked to in very little more time. The mention of deliberate exercise brings to the faces of many people a look of almost horror. Even with people who believe and accept the necessity for some positive action for the sake of their health and physical fitness, the will power is very often lacking and very half hearted efforts are all most of them manage.

It is no easier a task for these types of people to cut down their food intake. All too often the basic causes are psychological and the inability to handle their mental stresses goes hand in hand with their lack of resistance to overeating. Compulsive eating is very common, but as a means of relieving our mental tension and frustration it does little and merely adds to the sluggishness and inertia already prevailing. Cigarette smoking and alcohol consumption are also largely indulged in for similar escape although social drinkers would not be inclined to agree with this and smokers may say they wish to steady the nerves or some such alibi. When we are prepared to face this situation with honesty we are half way to being keen about doing something and further if we receive a mild or severe fright over the results of a medical examination, or perhaps suffer a coronary attack, then we are finally often forced to do something positive, give up smoking and heavy eating and take exercise.

The psychological attitude required to commence an exercise programme and restrictive diet is not really as difficult to acquire as many people fear. With the exercise itself the hardest part is the starting, the fear of what to many people is the unknown, brings out fears and inferiority complexes. They doubt their ability to do the exercises, they fear that they may look perhaps ridiculous and they may even fear or lack confidence in the courses prescribed or the instructor's method. Once over the initial hurdle, however, these fears vanish and the keenness grows as they progress and many become crusaders and teachers themselves. This attitude applies also to a change to more healthful eating habits and it comes as a surprise to many to discover that they no longer really desire the foods they once thought they could not live without. The actual shrinking of the stomach with fasting and light eating in itself is a great help because it results in a feeling of satiety with smaller amounts of food.

The problem of will-power really is basically one of firstly accepting without reservation the fact that today in our highly civilized living, health is not automatic. To be merely free of disease diagnosable by physicians and surgeons is not necessarily to be healthy and fit. Our unnatural living is not conducive to the health which blessed our primitive ancestors. They naturally had pure air, unspoiled food and were forced to work hard and fight for very existence. Further they frequently had fasting forced upon them. When we really accept this fact that we need to do something about our health then we are past our first hurdle.

The second fact to face up to is that what we are going to do is something that will need to be done for the rest of our lives, no three months health cure, then back to the old habits. We must realize fully also that permanent regular time must be kept for exercise. We can make this time more easily than we think. Do we not have to find time for bed when we are sick? Why wait until this happens. It also costs money to get sick. The final battle with our will power is perhaps not so easy to many because they may not believe that they can be much healthier. We need to constantly assure ourselves of the fact that the results are well worth the effort, to give ourselves a goal, to realize that the feeling of confidence that comes with mastery and control of our will is something very gratifying and quite frequently inspires us to further successes in all fields of endeavour. We need to talk with teachers, see examples, be inspired. All these boosts for strengthening our will power are available and we must seek them, use them and finally become such a boost ourselves for the help of our weaker brothers. Positive thinking works wonders and when weak in will, lacking in positive approach and action we must think ahead to what we are going to gain and not what we have to deny at the food table or the effort of exercise required. The exercise really becomes a pleasure after a while and the body really relishes it and looks for it. We can turn the fitness gained to good account in the playing of games, particularly in middle age, the winning of such games, the ego boost, that comes from beating our age group and even younger age groups. We feed our will-power with such thought, give ourselves the drive to progress, and gain health and happiness. We must condition our minds to the necessity of doing something about our health, strengthen our will-power and resolve to be firm and not fall for the easily forthcoming excuses such as lack of time, too tired, too busy and too old. The correct mental attitude is necessary and gives us such a flying start that success is just around the corner. Just as the battle to give up smoking is nearly half won when a person really deep down wants to give up, knowing the damage that can be done by continuing. Such people are usually so proud of their mastery and will-power that they find a new confidence in the ability to face life and hardships.

The psychological attitude and frame of mind must be cultivated and used to serve our needs for exercise whether it be for average health benefits or whether we need the intense mental dedication and fierce determination to be a world champion. Killer instinct, so necessary for champion class is born in many sportsmen and this psychological attribute is the one that makes one man train twice as hard to win. These types hate to lose and often figure in such fierce determined contests that they drive themselves past the pain barrier to reach the top. In many cases this type of psychological make-up can often carry a man or woman past the point of their skill limitation and enable them to beat persons of greater skill but with lesser psychological assets and qualifications.

Developing this attitude and trait is not easy. It is usually born with a personality. Some persons can have that basic design but have it latent under the surface of a well developed sense of fair play and brought out only if an opponent indulges in unfair tactics. We have all seen the fair player, patient and enduring, who has finally let go under the constant barrage of rough and dirty play. The mental make-up of a player not possessed of too great a skill is often a type of inferiority complex and a very large number of so called dirty players or rough, over vigorous players are cheats because of inferiority feelings over their skill lack. A highly skilled athlete in any sport does not have to resort to cheating, roughness or dirty tactics, he is capable of winning without and his confidence is boosted and kept high by the attitude of mind so possessed. He may be more honourable competing and losing but fairly than competing and winning by unfair tactics. Professionalism, of course, can change this attitude in some cases and the lure of money can often change a principle.

Mental attitude and approach to exercise can be very varied in different people and sex, but many excuses are common to all. It is all too easy to say we are busy, are fit enough and get enough exercise with the housework and in our jobs. We are never too busy and we are not fit enough and do not get sufficient exercise or the right type of exercise in our job. Even hard working labourers are often overweight. When a job entails hard physical effort it is not very long before we find an easy way to do it and a physically economical and saving way to do it. It becomes a bore and a monotonous drudge and does not have the pleasant recreational atmosphere necessary for best results. Nevertheless people engaged in hard work entailing movement are certainly far better off than a person sitting in an office all day, but they still can be better by indulging in games and recreational exercising.

Developing the mental approach, if one feels it lacking, may sometimes require quite a change in the pattern of daily living. Even if neuroses exist or states of anxiety above the normal prevail or even deep seated psychological problems are creating psychosomatic disorders we can obtain immense benefit by indulging in a healthy regime of living, with constant healthful thinking. The help of a psychiatrist should be sought and the advice followed and used to make the path smoother to realization of the necessity of action. We must realize that health does not easily come to us in our highly civilized manner of living —the stress is too great, the tension too tense, the competition too fierce. Mental disorders are on the increase and man has not yet evolved a resistance or natural counter to the stress and tension of modern life. We grow up with automation, the easy means of travel, the luxury of ample free time for pleasure and leisure. We pay the penalty for this and we must understand this. We must condition our thoughts and strengthen our will and resolve to do something about it or we will surely weaken further.

Our resolutions and our enthusiasm can be stimulated and fortified by constant contact and company of people who are examples of the healthful approach to life. We can exercise with them, under their guidance and above all within the atmosphere of enthusiasm that seems to radiate from such people. We should seek such people, learn from them and develop the attitude of mind to spur us to be a health enthusiast.

Mental attitude to defeat is an important factor in determining the amount of benefit we can obtain from games and competitive sport. The wrong attitude can even result in increased tension over a defeat or lack of form. A pleasant afternoon's golf with the objective in view of relaxing away from the office desk tension can finish up defeating the very purpose in playing, if the player's mental make-up is such that he or she cannot take defeat or a poor score card. If the blood pressure is raised by anger or frustration of one's poor showing and defeat, it is necessary to take stock of the mental approach or the results healthwise will not be what they are meant to be. One must keep in mind that the game is for the benefit of health and relaxation. It is no disgrace to be beaten and even champions go down at times. We must realize that the most important objective in playing sport and doing exercise is the improvement and building of health and fitness. The building of character is a feature also but this is even more constructive in defeat. Of course we all like to win and we should do our utmost to do so but if we are beaten by a better player we should adopt the attitude of seeking what we have learned in defeat.

For the person with the talent and skill to reach the top, dedication and sacrifice are two necessary characteristics. The dedication of the ballet dancer with the sacrifices of normal social pastimes is something not all dancers can endure. The self-denial of athletics and boxing and any other sport in which the inherent skill is obvious, is something very necessary. The realization that skill and natural physical assets are today not enough in themselves to lift a person to world class is an essential item in giving a person the spur and drive to train and practise. The mind is the master control and not enough is known yet of the wonderfully complex working of the brain or even less of the deep and complex psychology that it houses. The tremendous reserve of will that we possess is not anywhere near fully appreciated and this very will to win can be strong and fierce in some people to such a degree that they can overcome seemingly impossible handicaps to excel and reach the top. The rise of some boxers from the slums and poverty stricken childhood is an instance of the fighting qualities that are inherent in some people. Likewise racial under-privilege can produce its champions in spirit and determination.

For the person not concerned with the competition of sport, who merely wishes to exercise or play social games, the mental approach of a fierce will to win attitude is not so necessary perhaps, but there must be sufficiently strong purpose in mind so that whatever is undertaken is not done so with a lackadaisical approach resulting in very little exercise actually being done.

Further, we must enjoy what we are doing. Boredom results in early fatigue and we have *had* enough long before we have really *done* enough for any real benefit. Exercise routines must be done in pleasant surroundings and pleasant company. It must be varied and we must cultivate the psychological acceptance that we must do it and so make the best of it for best results. We must remember that our mind is a very powerful influence on our inclination whether or not to do something physical. How much easier it is to find the energy to do something we love doing such as dancing or swimming than to find it for some drudgery like household chores or humdrum work. We can be mentally tired long before we are physically worked out and the boredom of the long distance runner is a well known mental hurdle.

Many athletes and swimmers in training for long distance events have encountered this mental stagnation and have tried many ideas to overcome it and keep the mental drive so necessary for continuing. One of the most successful I have personally tried is the singing over in one's mind of a musical tune or humming, or imagining hearing it played by piano or orchestra. The tune can be in a time that would be suitable for ballroom dancing, particularly fox-trot rhythm; however, any tune or time would do so long as the tempo permits a foot touching the ground on the beat and inducing rhythm. Music has long been recognized as a spur and relief from fatigue. How often have we felt too tired for a walk but finish up going to a ball and dancing for miles. For swimming I have found a waltz time more suitable as this fits in more smoothly with the six beat crawl action of the legs.

The mental effort is greatly aided and much of the boring effect eliminated from long distance running by atmosphere and surroundings. New scenery, preferably countryside, engages our interest and new roads, bush tracks and country lanes keep us more alert for rough pathways, stumps, stones, etc. This occupation of our mental attention is very helpful in preventing the onset of staleness and fatigue which would come to us if running around a sports oval twenty to forty laps.

Probably the most important factor regarding the mental side of training is the realization and acceptance that it is with us and plays a very powerful part in our attitude, influencing not only our training and preparation but also our participation in sporting events. Even if we are exercising for health and fitness and not training specifically for a sport, we must accept the presence of psychological factors and constantly spur ourselves against disinclination and boredom. Monotonous routines should be varied, we must think out new variations, new exercises and even change sports, the latter more particularly as we get older and do not compete seriously. We must read, we must watch others, we must help and coach others, most particularly beginners. This gives us new interest and in fact gives us an added need to be fit and keep training ourselves. All these factors must be considered and used to help us maintain the drive and mental vitality so necessary to obtain the most benefit to our health. We must constantly remind ourselves that mental fatigue is very much more common and prevalent than actual physical fatigue. It is a very well proven fact that exercise done at home is never really very successfully done. Firstly it is mostly done alone, secondly it lacks the atmosphere. There are too many distractions, family, social, etc., and it is all too easy to be interrupted and put off. Whether we realize it or not, the strong driving force is missing and we almost invariably train less vigorously. Our mental attitude is weakened and finally we forget to do it and promise ourselves to do extra next time which incidentally we never do.

An important factor that also gives us relief from monotony is the playing of sport or exercising with the opposite sex; the recreational factor here makes light of the work whether the game or sport be lightly social or whether the members of the opposite sex be stars in women's sport and capable of giving one very serious competition and even beating the men in some cases.

The effect of spectator supporters for individuals or teams is very powerful in spurring on for victory, particularly in close finishes. If we have amongst the spectators our own families, loved ones and close friends, we have even further incentive to shine. The 'home territory' atmosphere also is worth points to our mental score in favour of producing our best or 'inspired best' which can be better than our best. We have all heard coaches say that our best will not be good enough and that we have to gear and spur our mental effort for a better best. We can do this, the will is there. We just have to master it, concentrate on it and use it to serve our needs with the call for greater physical effort.

The mind is a truly wonderful thing and we do not really know just what its limits are, if any, in influencing our body in normal daily functioning and when the demand for super physical effort is presented. Survival threat can bring out feats of endurance and stamina that are incredible and could never possibly be repeated again in ordinary athletic competition. Records are still being broken in all fields of sport. Where do they end, or do they end, why are we continuing to improve? It can be explained partly by greatly improved methods and knowledge regarding technique and nutrition but when the psychology of it all is weighed in, and we are trained or brainwashed to know that we can do a certain thing we are well and truly on the way to doing it. We do not know our capabilities and herein lies the most wide open field for research and new learning.

The magical influence of that wonder needle called confidence is something that we do not really fully understand. How different we feel, knowing we can do a thing, or can defeat a person because we have done it before, but how panicky and/or subdued we become if we, for an inexplicable reason, fail to do just this after having previously done it. What takes place in our mind that makes us apprehensive in our next attempt? What is the mysterious factor we call confidence? More important still as far as our future is concerned, how do we control it, how do we boost it, how do we use it for gearing our efforts to at least equal our best if not beat our best?

An important thought to hold in mind is that we have done it before, so therefore we *are capable* of it. We must resolve to train harder. Perhaps our fitness was suspect

Unless we are well past the age of athletic improvement we must remind ourselves that we do not go backwards— we must improve, so we must be capable of winning again. We must think, analyse, experiment and realize where we missed or failed, plan a different tactic, tell ourselves that we know we are better but just must make full use of our mental skill, and drive even further our physical capacity. This latter we seldom use to its fullest. We need not be afraid to push ourselves harder—we are made to stand terrific punishment and just so long as we know this, our confidence can rise just knowing that we have not used our fullest physical or mental resources. We must have confidence in the amazing forces of nature, our own physiology and the largely untapped mental powers and will that we have at our disposal.

I do not think it really wise or beneficial to excuse a temporary lapse with the thought that it was one of our off days or that we were just a bit unlucky. Whether or not this appeases our conscience is open to debate but no doubt exists about what it can do to our conscience and confidence. We cannot fool that part of our make-up and in fact we know if we are lying to ourselves. We know in our own hearts that we have not trained hard or strictly enough. We must accept the blame and resolve to dedicate our mind to a bigger effort and stricter self-denial. Our confidence rises as the severity of our training and discipline, and our conscience is clearer knowing that we have done our best. Remember that many a champion has been beaten by a fitter and better trained man even though he be less skilled. Boost your confidence by knowing that you trained better than ever before and you will surely thus do better than you have ever done before.

CHAPTER FIVE

Exercises for all
Needs for Men

The following exercise routines are intended to include or cover the needs of the youth, the middle-aged and the old-aged. They will include general health and tonic routines, development and general body building, and exercises of a nature conducive to the toning of bodily functions such as digestion, bowel and heart and lung. More specific treatment of internal malfunctioning will be included in the chapter on yoga as this ancient regime or system is concerned more with the health of the organs, the relaxation of the mind and nervous system.

The exercises are best done on an empty stomach and preferably late afternoon before the evening meal. Early morning pre-breakfast may also be suitable but I do not regard this time as satisfactory as the late afternoon. Some physiologies are at their peak in early morning whilst others—probably the majority—are evening peak types. Regularity is of prime importance—not necessarily regularity as regards the time of the day but of the days in the week. Two or three times is desirable with variations for weekend running or walking or the playing of games. They should be done with vigour and with the objective of sweating and puffing. As weather permits, clothing may be discarded to minimum and the exhilarating tonic effect of air on the body permitted. It is a sound precaution to be cleared of heart weakness, T.B., blood pressure or kidney disease and diabetes by medical check-ups. Some exercise may be done daily, whilst the full routine should be a 2–3 times weekly habit. The daily effort could be an early morning stretch out and deep breathing type, and more of a wake up stimulant to start the day. Muscle building routines of course can really only be done late afternoon or evening as they take more time and require longer rest periods between exercises.

In all routines the mental attitude must be positive, with confidence in the results; determination and perseverance must prevail, and patience possessed, for results of neglect over the years cannot be remedied in a few short weeks. Do not become mentally stale, vary the routines or order of the exercises, change days, work with others. Always if possible endeavour to use the fresh air, join a gym in preference to home venue, talk with fellow enthusiasts, compare, discuss improvement, and remember that what you are doing is what your body needs and was made to do for the maintenance of its efficiency and perfect health.

*Routines for the business and professional man—
suitable for tension and poor health generally*

(1) *Light warm up.* Run on the spot for a few minutes, wave arms around in circular motion backwards and forwards—stretch up and down.

(2) *Shoulder Circling.* Standing, arms bent with fists at shoulders, circle each shoulder up to ear, back, down, and forward in circling movement—10–15 times each shoulder —then 10 with both shoulders together.

(3) *Spine Flexion.* Clasp hands behind head, keeping legs almost straight, pull head to knees breathing out on the way down; return to upright whilst breathing in. Do 10–30 times and with reasonable speed and vigour.

(4) *Squats*. Standing with feet about 18 inches apart, heels flat, arms out frontwards, squat right down to sitting position—breathing out on way down and bounce up again breathing in. Heels should be kept flat throughout the whole movement. Start with 15 and work up to 50. Also increase tempo as fitness progresses. To assist breathing in, arms may be flung apart at shoulder level on the rebound up. May be done in sets of 2 or 3 with 30 reps.

(5) *Sit Ups*. Lying flat on floor, legs down straight, arms overhead, swing hands over to knees coming up to half sitting position, press on knees and breath out hard, return to lying position with arms overhead, breathing in as you go back. Next time over swing hands right to feet, breathing out on way down to feel, breathing in on way back to lying position. Alternate every second sit up to the feet. Commence with 10 repetitions and work up to 50. When sufficiently advanced you may do this on a sloping bench with feet up.

(6) *Knee fold ups*. Lying on back with hands clasped behind the head. Swing one knee up to the chest, lift head towards knee, but do not lift the body; breathe out as the knee is coming up. Straighten leg out and lower the head back breathing in as you do so. Alternate each knee coming up and do 15 with each knee. Rest a minute, then do same movement with both knees coming up together, raising head to meet them but keeping shoulders down on the floor. Begin with 10 and work up to 50. As in exercise 5 this can be done on abdominal sloping bench (feet down and head up) as fitness progresses.

(7) *To be done* only *after* progress has been such that exercise 5 is becoming easy. Lie on sloping abdominal board, feet up and secured, hands behind head, swing up with head towards knee, on the way up twist body twice to each side, return to lying position. Breath out on way up, in on way down. Commence with 5 repetitions

and work up to 10.

(8) *Back Arching.* Lying flat on floor face downwards, hands clasped over hips, lift body clear of the floor, breathing in on way up, lower down again breathing out. Begin with 10 and work up to 20. Progress to harder variation by doing on back arching bench or sloping board.

(9) *Push Ups.* Begin with 5 and work up to 20. Vary straight push ups with swooping through type. Do 2 or 3 sets of 10–15 repetitions.

(10) *Neck Exercise.* Bend head forward and backward —10 repetitions. Bend head to each side—10 each side. Turn head and look around over each shoulder—10 each shoulder. You can use the hand to offer mild resistance if desired. Circle head 3 times in each direction.

(11) *Breathing.* Standing, bend slightly forward, pressing hands together in front of thighs whilst breathing out hard (right out to the limit) keeping hands together stretch up to overhead whilst breathing in, hold breath and part the hands bringing arm down sideways to shoulder level, then breathe out and press hands together on front of thighs again. Do this exercise slowly and repeat 10 repititions.

(12) *Alternating running and squat.* 100 × 10—10 cycles. Run on spot for 100 counts, counting one as each foot touches the floor; on reaching 100 immediately go down to full squat on the ball of the foot, arms out straight in front of chest, and immediately bounce up again and do a small rebound in the upright position before going down to full squats—do 10—then commence 100 runs on spot again. This alternating cycle of 100 runs and 10 squats must be continuous and the squats must be on the ball of the foot, fast and rebounding. One set of 100 runs with 10 squats will be one cycle. Commence with 3 cycles and work up to 10 cycles as condition improves; as this exercise becomes easier, the pace should be pepped

up. You must always finish this exercise breathing quite heavily, so increase the tempo whenever possible to make you puff.

This whole routine should be done a minimum of twice weekly. At least twice a week on other days do a light steady jog or trot of 1–2 miles. In addition to this routine of exercises you are advised to do some of the Yoga poses and the breathing daily. Study the chapter on Yoga, particularly the relaxation technique and practise it daily. Do the Yoga routine at least 3 times weekly, alternating your exercise routine.

The Yoga Asanas you should do are numbers 1, 2, 4, 7, 8 and 10.

Follow the diet principles outlined in Chapter 3 on Nutrition, be particularly strict in avoiding animal fats and *do not smoke*. Include in your diet daily a salad with plenty of lettuce, raw cabbage and carrots. Take maintenance dosage of natural vitamin E and C and at least one teaspoon of molasses daily, also one desertspoonful of powdered brewer's yeast. Use a lecithin preparation daily or twice daily and eat soya beans in preference to meats as often as practicable. Take 1 teaspoonful of cider vinegar and one of honey in glass of warm water on retiring. Get plenty of sunbathing or alternatively take sunlamp baths. Have occasional Sauna baths, and a dry or infrared irradiation cabinet, have cool or cold showers in preference to hot baths. Sleep in fresh air as much as available, take long walks and enjoy dancing.

Do not be content with mere negative health. There is a vast difference being merely free from diagnosable complaints and being really radiantly healthy and alive with vitality and stamina.

Positive radiant health is possible in a highly civilized

state of existence only by positive effort. The factors working against natural, vital health are too many. We need to do something to counteract the ill effects of polluted air, denatured food and the lazy habits brought about by the modern comforts of present day living. We must exercise and exercise plenty, we must study the food we eat and partake only that which is unrefined not preserved, not artificially coloured and overcooked. We must think health, seek it and go get it and hold it, it is the most priceless possession we'll ever have. All too often it is only fully appreciated when we begin to lose it.

The exercise routine for the older person, man or woman should be done very slowly and easily at first beginning with 5–6 repetitions and working up steadily. Do not do all of the exercises and any that are to difficult, leave until stronger and fitter. Perseverence and regularity are necessary. Do not allow yourself to become distressed. Do the Yoga poses, read the Yoga chapter thoroughly, practise the breathing and especially Savasana Relaxation.

Exercises of Elementary Routines for development and body building

Recommended for the youth but can be done by middle aged under guidance and supervision and in restricted manner regarding number of sets and repetitions and total time of work-out.

Apparatus required will be dumbells and barbells. Advanced variations and routines will not be included here as these require extensive apparatus, pulleys, leg press machines, lat machines, etc., which are well catered for in modern gymnasiums. Further, a few isometrics will be included as an adjunct to the weight resistant exercises for each muscle group. Isometrics does not entail movement or apparatus work, so could be used more extensively if the apparatus is not available. It would not be possible to do all of the exercises for each muscle group and to do each muscle group in any one work-out. It is suggested that you note the muscles and muscle groups in most urgent need for your building and do these exercises to cover what muscles you select. Three times weekly is the average number of work-outs for most people but you can arrive at your own limitations by experiment. Some will be capable of 4–6 work-outs per week, others will be used up by twice weekly work-outs.

Be guided by how you feel fronting up for each work-out, keeping in mind the difference between laziness and muscle fatigue from too frequent work-outs. Watch your weight, signs of fatigue and lack of appetite.

Although each muscle group series of exercises will be specifically for that group of muscles in particular, other muscles will be brought into the exercise as minor auxiliary workers also, and much overlapping will occur but this of course is all for the better and is perfectly natural the way the body is mechanically constructed and will ensure against strain and possible dislocation. It is advised that an anatomical atlas be obtained to facilitate the learning of muscle names and location and function.

In all the following progressive weight resistance exercises the weight should be increased whenever possible regularly.

Shoulder Girdle Area

(1) Hold dumbells in front of thighs, backs of hands facing out. Swing straight arms up overhead breathing in, down again and breathing out. Do 10–15 repetitions. Can be varied by doing arms alternately. Hold dumbells on side of thighs, backs of hands facing outward, swing up sideways breathing in, down again breathing out. 10–15

repetitions. Use dumbells of sufficient weight to ensure that 8th, 9th and 10th repetitions are a bit of a struggle without using body swing to help. Repeat for 3 sets.

(2) Hold dumbells at shoulder level. Press each dumbell up to arm's length and down alternately. 10–15 repetitions, and then both together for 5 repetitions. Breathe in on way up and out on way down. Use sufficient weight, repeat for 3 sets.

(3) Barbell presses behind neck. Hold barbell behind neck and press to arm's length overhead, breathing in on way up and out on way down. If available, a bent bar is preferable. Do 10 repetitions and sufficient weight to make it a struggle for the 10th repetition. Do 3 sets.

These last 2 exercises will give considerable movement to the triceps muscle on the back of the upper arm, also the trapezius in back and neck.

Upper arm—flexor—biceps and brachialis routines

(1) Dumbell curls. Hold dumbells in front of thighs, backs of hands against thighs—keeping elbow firmly against hip, curl dumbell up to shoulder and lower down again. Repeat with other arm. Do 10 repetitions with each arm. Rest and repeat for 3 sets of 10 repetitions.

(2) Same position as exercise 1, but using barbell. Same movement, 10 repetitions and repeat for 3 sets of 10 repetitions.

(3) Lean over sloping bench from the top and lay the arm down along bench, curl dumbell up to shoulder. Repeat 3 sets of 10 repetitions with each arm.

Back—Upper and Lower

(1) *Bowing Exercise.* Stand with barbell or dumbell on back of neck. Bend forward bringing head to knees, breathing out, return to upright breathing in. Begin with light

weight and work up gradually, do not jerk and make sure that you are well warmed-up first. Lower back strain must be watched for and care is needed. Do 3 sets of 10 repetitions.

(2) *Bent over Rowing Motion.* Bend over to a position with legs straight and trunk parallel to floor, preferably with forehead resting on a bench or against wall. Hold barbell hanging down at arm's length and pull it into chest and lower. Do 3 sets of 10–12 repetitions.

(3) *Dead Lift* with legs straight. Keeping legs straight, bend body over and grasp barbell, straighten up till barbell is against thighs, breathing in, lower, and breathe out. Take care here, *do not jerk* and begin with very light weight and work up with gradual increases. Do 3 sets of 10 repetitions. When well advanced after 2 to 3 months, you can use heavy weight for less repetitions as 5 sets of 5.

(4) *Chin Ups.* Do 3 sets of the maximum number of repetitions you can do. If a lat machine is available do 3 sets of 8 to 10 with heavy weights. This exercise also gives considerable movement to the arm muscles. Can be done with palms to front and/or palms facing in.

Abdominal

(1) Sit ups on abdominal bench with weight behind head. Begin with light weights and work up gradually. Do 3 sets of 10–20 repetitions, after 10–15 weeks, occasional variation with heavy weight for 5 sets of 5 repetitions.

(2) Vary with twisting sit ups.

Legs, Thighs and Calves

(1) Squats or deep knee bends. Use bent bar for preference. Feet about 12–15 inches apart, heels on low board (about 1–2 inches high). Keep back straight and go down to full squat, and return to upright. Breathe in before going down and hold breath on way down and up, breathing out

just before fully straightening the knees. Do 3–5 sets of 10–20 repetitions. Can be varied or alternated with half knee bends going down half way.

(2) Leg press machine if available do 3–5 sets of 10–20 repetitions.

(3) Iron Boot Routine. Using iron boot if available or bag of sand strapped to foot, sit on high bench or table with lower leg dangling down and thigh resting on table. Straighten leg out and tighten knee strongly. Use fairly heavy weight and do 5 sets of 10–15 repetitions. An excellent exercise for cartilage damage and the restoration of thigh after cartilage removal surgery.

(4) Using iron boot, keep whole leg straight and raise stiff and straight out in front as in dancers high kick—3 sets of 10 repetitions.

(5) Using barbell on neck, rise up and down on toes keeping knees straight, do 3 sets of 10–15 repetitions more beneficial if done with toes on block of wood and starting with heels down.

(6) Sit in full squat position, rise up and down on toes lifting heels, whilst staying in squat position.

Chest Routine

D.B. Circling on bench

(1) Lying flat on back on bench, take dumbells, hold together at arm's length above chest—keeping D.B. together, lower back overhead parallel to floor, part and swing round horizontally to the thighs bringing together over the thighs and continue circle back again to overhead. Maintain a continuous circling movement, breathing in deeply as you swing back overhead and out strongly as you swing round to the thighs. Do 3 sets of 10.

(2) *Bench Press.* Lying on bench take barbell and hold at arm's length over chest (if available use bent bar). Take

a deep breath, hold breath and lower bar to chest, do not stop but straighten out again to arm's length over chest, breathe out just as the arms are straightening out. Do 5 sets of 8–12 repetitions and endeavour to increase weight regularly, or whenever able, at the rate of 10 lb. increases.

This exercise is one of the best upper body developers and brings in the triceps and anterior deltoid as well as being an excellent chest developer both for the pectoral muscles and the depth of the thorax generally.

(3) *Straight arm and bent arm pullovers on bench.* Lying on back on bench, hold weight at arm's length over chest (you can use a barbell or centrally loaded dumbell) take a very deep breath and lower weight straight out overhead, breathe in, and return to arm's length over chest. Do 3 sets of 10. *Caution:* Do *not* have elbows completely locked. Same position with close grip, hands nearer to each other, lower down with elbows well bent and return on chest. 3 sets of 10.

(4) Lie on bench, on back, hold heavy dumbells at arm's length with a slight bend at the elbow lower until slightly below, parallel to the floor, taking in a deep breath as you are lowering down. Return to position above chest, breathing out as you do so. Do 3 sets of 10. This exercise can also be done on a sloping bench. No specific exercise will be given here to the backs of the upper arm, the triceps muscle, as this muscle gets a work-out in the 2nd and 3rd exercise for the shoulder girdle area (see page 72), and further with the bench or supine press exercise (see page 74).

Neck Exercises

If head harness neck exerciser is not available, excellent neck exercise can be had by doing the wrestlers' bridge using wide range of movement. Lie on back and arch up so that you are on the top of your head and heels. Rock backwards and forwards and up and down—10–20 repetitions. It is not intended in the scope of this book to go further into development routines as much apparatus would be needed. Any body builder wishing to go further would need to join a gymnasium and would have coaching and instruction available in such a place.

In addition to the body building training, a jog or run of 2–3 miles, should be taken at least once weekly, depending on energy available after heavy weight exercises. These latter do not provide the cardio-pulmonary, vascular system with as beneficial a work-out as is desirable, so the inclusion of a run should be a weekly or twice weekly event. Aim at getting the pulse rate down in the low 60s at least.

Take pulse check after weight exercises routine and compare with check taken. 2–3 hours after a good run, even the next morning after the run.

Isometrics

Isometric exercise has the very desirable and useful advantage of being able to be done almost anywhere and in almost any position, or situation. It can be done sitting, standing, lying, sitting at the office desk, or in the motor car; it requires no apparatus and very little time. You can invent your own exercises as you go along once you know the basic principle and with a little elementary knowledge of anatomy you could map out a whole programme to cover the entire body. Very little space other than that which your body itself occupies, is needed, and movement is not necessary. A mere few seconds per day can increase your strength amazingly, in some cases doubling it in a very short space of time. The basic principle of isometric exercise is that of tensing a muscle against a resistance that does not yield. Maximum muscle contraction is induced, as no movement takes place, the unyielding resistance bringing about a greater call of muscle fibres into action. The length of time for holding this tension of muscle need be only as short as 5–6 seconds for the overall increases in strength to be as much as 5% over a very few days or so. Isometric exercise can be spread out over the day using the different positions of the body during the day for different muscle contractions and areas. For instance, whilst sitting in a chair, you can grasp the underneath of the chair each side with the hands and endeavour to lift the chair whilst still sitting in it. You will not move the chair one inch but you will get a powerful muscle tension trying to do so.

The following list of isometric exercises although intended to be merely a guide can give you a fairly comprehensive work-out and increase your overall strength. Most of the body's voluntary muscles will be used, but once you know the main principle you can invent your own exercises by just tensing a muscle and endeavouring to move something that does not yield. You must not jerk, but push or pull steadily and as strongly as able for a mere 5 or 6 seconds. It is not meant to suggest that isometrics take the place of general training, but more as a supplement and adjunct to it. Movement is necessary for heart and lung benefits, isometrics is more specifically a muscle strengthener rather than a constitutional tuning. Nevertheless constitutional benefits will be noticed particularly with the strengthening and firming up of the abdominal muscle wall with subsequent internal organic toning up.

Each of these exercises will cover a different muscle or group and from the basic idea you can work out more variations for any particular muscle needs:

(1) Place hand against side of head push strongly but do not allow the head to move—resist—hold 5 seconds. Do the

same with other hand on other side.

(2) Standing in doorway, place back of hands against sides of doorway push out with full power (trying to widen doorway) hold for 5 seconds.

(3) Standing in doorway, palms against sides of doorway, press out again with full power hold 5 seconds.

(4) Place hands with palms up against top of doorway, push up hold 5 seconds.

(5) Standing side-on in doorway, place palms each side of door and press in strongly hold 5 seconds.

(6) Standing leg straight, bend down and grasp feet under the arches, try hard to pull the feet off the floor hold 5 seconds.

(7) Standing in doorway, hands pressed against top of doorway with *arms straight*, knees bent. Keep arms straight and endeavour to straighten knees hold 5 seconds.

(8) Lying face downwards, feet held firmly under heavy furniture keeping legs straight, try to lift the furniture with legs hold 5 seconds.

(9) Lying on back, legs straight, feet secured down, hold a heavy weight behind head, hold arms under heavy furniture, tense the abdominal muscles by attempting to sit up hold tight for 5 seconds and then relax.

(10) Stand against a heavy table, place elbow firmly against hip, and wrist under the table edge, try to curl the forearm up without any other movement of the arm. The table must be heavy enough to be immovable by one arm, hold 5 seconds and repeat with other arm.

You can go on from here with countless variations for any muscle, or group of muscles, by improvising and utilizing any objects; furniture, even your car at each traffic stop, grip your steering intensely for 5 seconds, then relax, push back hard against your seat 5 seconds then relax. By keeping in mind the basic principle of trying to move an unyielding resistance you can, by tensing for

5 seconds or so, give the muscles a thorough full fibre work-out.

The following is an advanced type of alternating run and squat routine very suitable and beneficial for footballers and any other sport where leg bounce and stamina are required. It will improve leaping agility, and will greatly speed up take off power for sports where acceleration and short dashes are the prime necessities. It is calculated on an ascending and descending scale basis and consists of alternating runs on the spot with bouncing fast squats done with a little rebound at the top of the squat finish.

It is advisable that this advanced version of alternating run and squat routine be attempted only when fitness has reached a stage capable of handling it. It is suggested that you *not* go fully up the scale to the 100 runs × 30 squats level for a few weeks and do not stay on the same level for 3 cycles as outlined on the scale until quite able to maintain breathing power and leg bounce.

When able to go up the scale, and able to do 3 cycles at the top before returning down the scale, you will have reached excellent fitness and have very good staying power. Progress from here would be a matter of shortening your time, so when the scale becomes within your power to complete, aim at decreasing the time taken, pep up your pace. After descending down the scale to the 50 runs × 5 squats do a very fast finishing sprint of 100 runs on the spot. Athletes competing in sports requiring sprint runs, jumps, hurdles, etc., will find this an excellent builder. Adding knee-chest jumps completes the routine as a fine all round leg and wind conditioner.

Commence with:	50 runs	followed by		5 squats
immediately followed by:	60 ,,	,,	,, 10	,,
	70 ,,	,,	,, 15	,,
	80 ,,	,,	,, 20	,,
	90 ,,	,,	,, 25	,,
	100 ,,	,,	,, 30	,,
	100 ,,	,,	,, 30	,,
	100 ,,	,,	,, 30	,,
	90 ,,	,,	,, 25	,,
	80 ,,	,,	,, 20	,,
	70 ,,	,,	,, 15	,,
	60 ,,	,,	,, 10	,,
	50 ,,	,,	,, 5	,,

CHAPTER SIX

Health, Fitness and
Beauty for Women

When discussing and mapping out exercise routines for ladies, it must be kept in mind that prime importance is attached by the ladies themselves to the beauty and youthful appearance value of any programme. With many ladies it is quite an incidental side effect and fringe benefit that this same programme will also considerably improve their health and vitality. In actual fact the health is bound up with the beauty and youth, and it is virtually impossible to remain looking young and beautiful for very long if the health and fitness are lacking. The skin, the hair, the eyes, the posture, even the walk are all give-aways regarding age. A youthful body kept firm and shapely by exercise, a healthy skin kept so by vital diet, a clear eye by the same diet, all are treasured possessions and assets in the battle to stay younger by being healthier.

It is desirable that the programme outlined in this chapter be carefully and conscientiously followed and adhered to as a pattern of living, and not merely as a crash programme for a short time. Health and youthful beauty are bound up and dependent on daily practice of healthful living for the rest of the long life that is within reach. A habit must be established of doing things the healthy, exercising way, and not the lazy way, of eating the healthful and youth-preserving foods instead of the devitalized, vitamin deficient foods so prevalent. The greater use of cold water and fresh air on the skin should be encouraged, and less of the luxuriant indulgence in hot soapy baths.

The best results from this programme will be obtained if the chapter on Yoga is carefully studied and the Asanas and breathing exercises therein regularly practised. Yoga is a wonderful relaxer, and the ability to relax is a decided asset in the preservation of youthful looks, health and beauty. Yoga is further an excellent system for improving the health and efficiency of the internal organs, also the flexibility of the spine and body generally. Above all, it can bring to the mind the peaceful outlook and ability to handle problems and remain calm, serene and happy, free from tension and worry.

An excellent combination of this programme and that outlined in Chapter 7 would be that of 2–3 sessions weekly of each. If time is a problem, remember that time is what is creeping up on you, so go to it and use it with a priority on something which is going to defer the very ravages that time itself is bringing. Even if you do a mere 15 minutes daily of the important exercises and Yoga poses, results will be gratifying and rewarding.

The exercise routine should be done in its entirety at least twice a week, and some of the stretching and Yoga poses done daily. Some, more particularly the breathing and stretching, may be done early morning pre-breakfast, and the relaxing practised in the evening, but in all of these, individual preferences and variations—depending on personal physiology and circumstance—are permissible with regard to time of day and the exercises chosen. They must be performed, however, with vigour, and if weight reduction is sought, must be done for longer until detectable perspiration level is reached.

The diet needs to be adjusted to the right calorie level intake, and a calorie chart kept handy for ready reference.

the health value of foods must be kept in mind, and the value of certain foods for skin beauty realized. Tobacco is an enemy not only of the heart and lungs and blood vessels, but of the skin and eyes, and smoking should be completely avoided. Even smoky atmospheres should, whenever possible, be avoided. Moderation in alcohol consumption is advisable, as it is not necessary or in any way beneficial or helpful to the preservation of good looks and youth. The so-called stimulation or kick is really non-existent. No bodily functions are really improved by the consumption of alcohol. We merely feel that they are, with that false security of inhibitory release.

The following exercises will cover the needs of the whole body for general health, suppleness, shape and firmness. More exercises for the hips, thighs and abdomen will be included, as these areas are the problem spots for most women. They can be used by all ages and sizes. The amount done, the number of repetitions of each exercise, will be dependent on the needs regarding reducing. The age must be also taken into consideration, and it is wise to begin steadily and increase the vigour as fitness increases. Those wishing to reduce must do more repetitions of each exercise. They will also, of course, need to follow a low calorie diet in conjunction with the exercise programme. It is advisable, also, that a long vigorous walk of 2–3 miles be taken as often as possible—at least three times weekly.

In addition, any games such as tennis or golf should be taken up as an added calorie output and mental variety. Weekly or bi-weekly steam baths would also be a help. In fact, anything which calls for activity, produces sweating and generally keeps a woman physically busy, should be indulged in if wishing to reduce. Boredom must be strictly avoided because of its psychological side effect—compulsive eating. Likewise, frustration, repression and such must be eliminated, as they too can lead to eating as an escape compensation.

Exercises suitable for girls and women for health, fitness and figure

(1) Warm up with some running on the spot for about 3 or 4 minutes.

(2) Stand with feet apart, arms out sideways from the shoulders; begin circling the arms backwards alternately as in backstroke swimming, use body sway and have knees slightly bent. Do vigorously for a minimum of 20 each arm —work up to 50 each arm. (Shoulders, back and waist.) Fig. 1.

(3) *Spine bends.* Stand with feet about 2–2½ feet apart, hands behind head. Breathing out, pull head down to R knee, return to upright breathing in, continue to L knee the same. Do 15 to each knee, then 10 between knees. Increase to 25 each knee if desired. Fig. 2.

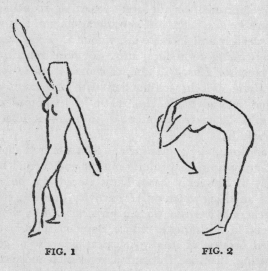

FIG. 1   FIG. 2

(4) *Squats.* Stand with feet about 12 inches apart, arms in front straight out. Keep heels flat and squat right down, returning vigorously to upright. Breathe out on way down, breathe in on way up. Begin with 15 repetitions and work up to 30. If reducing is required for heavy thighs, repeat this for 3 sets of repetitions. (For legs and hips.) Fig. 3.

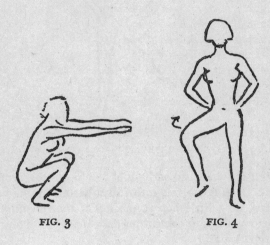

FIG. 3   FIG. 4

(5) *Hip circumduction.* Stand on one leg (hold on to wall or chair if balance difficult, but endeavour to do without support. Raise other knee bent up to waist level in front, circle knee in a backward direction around and out, and return to front. Do from 20–40 repetitions, then change leg. (For hips and hip joints.) Fig. 4.

(6) *Side kicks.* Stand with feet together, hands on hips, swing one leg out and sideways as high as possible, vigorously, and return. Do between 20–30 repetitions and repeat with other leg. Do 2 or 3 sets of this if thigh is thick on the outside and hips heavy on the sides. Fig. 5.

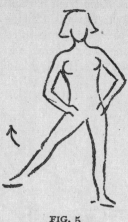

FIG. 5

(7) *Fast squats.* Stand on balls of feet or on toes, arms out in front. Drop down fast into full squat and rebound up again fast, do a little hop at the top of the rebound, and straight down again, continuing fast and with vigour. Do 20–30 repetitions.

(8) Stand with feet about 6 inches apart with toes turned in, heels turned out, rise up and down on toes as high as possible and do 10 repetitions; then turn toes out and heels in as in ballet position, do same rising on toes and down—10 repetitions.

Stand with weight on outside of heels with toes and front of foot more or less off the floor, roll foot from the outside of the heels to the inside, and reverse. Do 10 repetitions. (For the calves and ankles.)

(9) Standing on one leg, swing the other one forward as high as possible, then right through backwards as high back and up as possible. Do vigorously and at least 20 with

each leg—increase to 40 or more if desired. (For the front of thigh and back of hips.) Fig. 6.

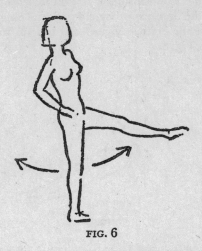

FIG. 6

(10) *Sit Ups and Twist*. Lying on back, feet about 2½ feet apart, thumbs locked, swing up and over with both hands to one foot, breathing out; return to lying position, breathing in. Then repeat to other foot. Swing head close to the knee as you come over. Do 15 to each knee, and increase to 25 each knee if waist and abdomen flabby and bulky. Fig. 7.

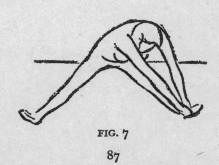

FIG. 7

(11) Sit up with legs out in front straight, arms back behind with hands resting on floor. Lift hips off floor, twist body and bounce side of hip on floor, then twist the other way and bounce other side of hip on floor. Do as fast as you can, bounce vigorously and do minimum of 20 each side. Fig. 8.

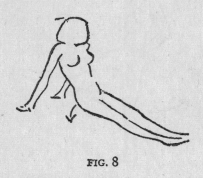

FIG. 8

(12) Sit on floor with legs out straight, arms at shoulder level with elbows bent. Swivel and twist hips and body forward across floor as fast as possible, then repeat same going backwards. Try to push each leg and hip forward as far as possible, then swivel and twist the other leg and hip forward, and so on. Do at fast rate and do 2–3 laps across room. (For hips and waist.)

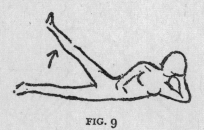

FIG. 9

(13) Lying on side, swing top leg up as high as it will go, and down. Do 15–25, then change sides and do other leg. Then do same raising both legs together, ankles touching, and do 10 each side. Try to keep body and legs in a straight line. Fig. 9.

(14) Lying on back, hands behind head, legs straight down, fold alternate knee to chest, pulling head to meet knee. Do 15 to 20 each knee, then 10–15 with both knees coming up. Breathe out as folding up; breathe in as straightening out. (Abdomen and thighs.) Fig. 10.

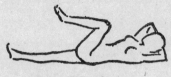

FIG. 10

(15) Same position as (14). Do scissor kicks up and down, and sideways. Do as many as 10–15 if possible. (Abdomen and thighs.)

(16) Lie on floor on back, arms stretched out sideways from shoulders, hold something heavy in hands; fold both knees up on to chest, roll both knees over to floor on one side and swing them right across chest to floor on the other side. Do 15 to each side and increase to 20 if waist requires it. (For the waist.) Fig. 11.

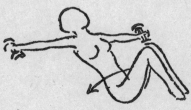

FIG. 11

(17) Lying face downwards, arms out in front, raise each leg alternately as high as possible. 10–20 repetitions. (For the hips and back.)

(18) On hands and knees. Lower chin down to floor between hands, and as the chin is going down begin swinging a leg out straight and upwards; return leg and push up from floor until on hands and knees position again. Alternate each leg going out and up as the chin goes down each time. Do 25 with each leg; do as fast as possible and push up hard from floor, straightening arms. (For the hips and back; also an excellent bust exercise.) Fig. 12.

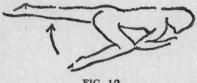

FIG. 12

(19) Same position as (18)—i.e. on hands and knees. Keeping *arms* perfectly *straight*, swing head under and swing R knee under abdomen, then swing knee and straighten out leg up high and back with plenty of back arch, at the same time swinging head up and back, to create an arch from heel to back of head. Swing both head and knee

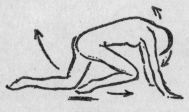

FIG. 13

90

under body again, keeping the swing going under and out continuously for 30 repetitions with each leg. Start slowly, and as the technique is mastered work up to a very vigorous tempo. (For the back, hips and thighs.) Fig. 13.

(20) Lying face downwards, secure feet firmly under chair, sofa or something to hold them; clasp hands behind head, arch back and lift body as high as possible, breathing in on way up and out on way down. 10–20 repetitions. (For the back.) Fig. 14.

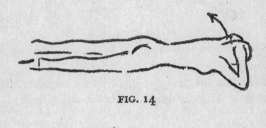

FIG. 14

Exercises specific for bust development and contouring

Exercises for bust development must aim at increasing the circulation into and through the muscles beneath the bust, and also into the bust itself. Improved depth of thorax is a desirable adjunct in the appearance of the bust. Massage is also useful, particularly in conjunction with the exercise.

(A) Dumbell circles on bench. Lie flat on back on a bench, hold dumbells together at arm's length above chest; keeping together, lower dumbells back over head until arms are parallel to floor, part the arms and swing the dumbells around sideways down to the side of the thighs, bring together over the thighs and swing straight back over the head again. Keep this movement going in a continuous circle, breathing in as you swing back overhead, breathing out as you swing dumbells around to thighs. Do 3 sets of 15 repetitions. Fig. 15.

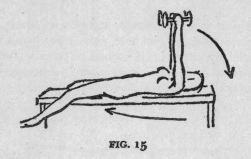

FIG. 15

(B) Do exercise (18).

(C) Standing up straight, place palms together over the bust level or slightly higher, elbows out sideways. Push

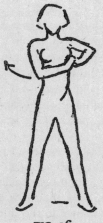

FIG. 16

one hand strongly across to one side and then push back across to other side, resisting strongly each time with one hand, whilst pushing with the other. Do 10–15 to each side, and resist strongly with one hand each time. Fig. 16.

Massage may be done between each exercise, and consists of lightly grasping the bust in the palm of the hand with fingers spread out wide around it. Move the bust itself around in circling movements over the underlying pectoral muscle. Do at least 20 circles in each direction. Next move the entire hand and fingers over the bust itself, moving mostly in an upward direction. An added benefit is to dip the hands in cold water, and splash on the bust with the massage movements.

Finish with deep breathing for 5–10 breaths. Make the breathing slow and stretch the arms upwards high as you breathe in, press hands together firmly in front of thighs as you breathe out.

As will be seen after reading these 20 exercises, many overlap each other in the type of movement and area of body worked on. This can provide variation, and you can pick out any 2 or 3 for each area and do, and change every few weeks if desired. It is advisable, however, to do abdominal exercises in all routines for health value, and pick out as many of the rest for hips and legs as your type of body needs, or where any obesity exists.

The importance of correct eating for health, beauty and youthful appearance cannot be too strongly emphasized. The benefits of the exercises are enhanced to considerable length if diet is watched and controlled for nutritious value as well as calorific restriction. A calorie chart is necessary for your handy reference. For what not to eat, and the list from which to choose your health giving foods, refer to the lists in Chapter 3 on Nutrition. Here are the foods you must include daily for health, and which will give you a clear bright eye, shiny hair, and a lovely skin:

All fresh fruits in season, salad vegetables—especially carrot—cucumber, raw cabbage, lettuce, celery and tomatoes. Have at least one teaspoonful of molasses, honey, powdered brewer's yeast, cider vinegar (in glass of water) sometime during the day. Eat only pure wholemeal bread, and very sparingly if weight watching, drink herb teas and avoid coffee and tea; learn to live without the fatal fag, if already a smoker. Drink only water if thirsty, and, if you can get it—distilled water.

Also to your daily diet add natural Vitamin E tablets and natural Vitamin C compounds, if there is any doubt as to vitamin sufficiency. Eat only grilled meats, and frequently use soya beans as meat substitute. Do not drink pasteurised milk, but yoghourt or buttermilk in moderation may be eaten or drunk—plain and without artificial or synthetic fruit flavouring. Avoid all fried foods, greasy mixtures and roasts, chocolates, cakes and sugary desserts, and ice cream.

Do as much walking in clean, bush air or countryside as you can, and include dancing as recreational pastime. Use cold water plentifully on your face and rub vigorously; do not use soap, even the mildest; have cool showers and rub with towel until glowing; avoid heavy make-up; a beautifully healthful skin requires no adjunct or adornments—health is your best make-up.

Exercises for the sportswomen must necessarily be of a more athletic nature, and will need to include a certain amount of weight resistance movements, as strength must be considered in the developmental training for anybody, male or female. As the basic strength building exercises vary very little when it comes to sport training, the women athletes may do very much the same routine as the men, but on a modified scale. The arm and chest routines may be done by the women javelin and discus throwers, whilst sprinters may benefit from the thigh and calf routines. I would not advise, however, that heavy weighted squat exercises be done by the women, but rather to use the leg press. High jumpers and broad jumpers will need the basic leg strengthening routines, and will also obtain much benefit from including the alternate running and squat routine of the advanced type. For this refer to Chapter 5.

Swimmers should use the chest routine exercises, and in addition add the pulley weight exercises, standing and lying along a bench.

Team sports, such as hockey and softball, cricket and basket ball, all require solid leg work, and plenty of early season running of 2–3 miles, or even more. Fast, squat movements with rebound, and 2–3 times weekly the alternate running and squat routine should be done, particularly the advanced one of ascending and descending scale as outlined in Chapter 5. For softball, the chest and waist routines must be done, and also plenty of half squat movements, to improve base work and throwing power. Push ups should be done for 5–10 repetitions and for 2–3 sets. Back arching routines on the sloping bench should also be included.

Do not allow yourself to become overweight. The diet must be restricted and health foods consumed in preference to starchy refined ones. Count the calories and your stamina will be increased. Excess weight adds strain to heart and lungs, with consequent decrease in endurance. Women athletes can, contrary to some opinions, avoid the hefty masculine look. Femininity need not be lost by being an athlete, but can sometimes be enhanced by the grace and beautiful movement developed.

Although dedication is required to reach the top, and much of the social whirl and activity must be foregone, the woman athlete does not necessarily have to be so different. Social pastime should be encouraged, dancing and other recreational pursuits should be indulged in as a happy diversion for relaxation. Whatever sport is played, women should walk more often. Organized hikes are ideal for the social atmosphere, and also as a hip exercise to keep this area slim and trim, because bulk and weight gain seem so easily come by in this area.

Marriage and motherhood need not be deferred. In most cases it can work for the better, as a more settled sex life and fuller maturing of a woman's physiology become developed. Happiness and freedom from tension are both constructive factors for fitness. Time should be found for reading and general mental exercise with thought-provoking topics. Balance is important.

CHAPTER SEVEN

Yoga

Yoga is almost surely the most ancient of regimes for the practice of healthful living. It has today so many ramifications that nobody could hope to learn them all. The basic principles, however, are all the same, and the Asanas, or exercise poses, are all found in Yoga beginning. The Hatha Yoga, with which we will be dealing here, is primarily the elementary phase of purification of the body through Asanas and breathing. This will be found the objective and the reasons that the largest number of people take up Yoga. Anybody wishing to go further after mastering Hatha Yoga, to practice the Raja and spiritual, will need to have a trained teacher; it is not sufficient to read from a book.

Probably no greater or more successful system exists for relaxing than Yoga. The breathing and relaxation techniques are proven and regular, and conscientious practice will bring results that can change the whole outlook and temperament. I have seen bad-tempered, worrying types of personality change to placid, pleasant and sincerely happy and confident ones.

The very nature of Yoga and the production of such temperament is one of the reasons that Yoga is considered, and in fact is, the most youthifying of all physical culture systems. The preservation of youth and beauty is a tremendous advantage as the years pass by us, and we have the increased knowledge and wisdom that comes with age, plus the retaining of youthful looks and physical vigour. The suppleness and flexibility of the spinal column, and the body generally, is a factor in the excellent posture of people doing Yoga. The effect of certain Asanas on the circulation to various organs is to greatly improve the function of these organs. The improved digestion and bowel function is a prime factor in the overall gain in health that Yoga brings. Further to the circulatory improvement is the effect of a greatly stimulated flow of nervous energy to the organs by the spinal toning that Yoga gives, and pinched discs, nerve pressures are quite frequently freed. Lumbago and the family of rheumatic, fibrositic pains so commonly suffered by the large majority of people are non-existent among the faithful Yoga adherents. Many disorders just simply disappear after a few months of regular practice of Yoga Asanas and breathing.

Yoga, however, is not merely a system of exercise Asanas and breathing with advanced spiritual meditation, but is more an overall method of living. Diet followed is simple and non-stimulating, and the avoidance of certain foods and substances is advised. It is quite akin to Nature Cure principles, and many Yogis advise against the taking of drug treatments for ailments. Removal of the basic cause of disease and adherence to natural principles is a feature of Yoga teaching, and in fact a feature of true physical culture teaching.

Yoga preaches non-violence, non-greed, non-lust and non-injury. It preaches the observance of the golden rule as we know it, and preaches the practice of clean body, clean mind, with the spiritual attainment of reality with the Supreme Universal Being. It teaches the love of God, but does not insist that you change the religion through which you worship God, but that you realize the existence and power of the Almighty Being and observe.

This chapter of this book is not to be a comprehensive

one on Yoga, but merely an introductory lesson for beginners. Many good books are available that go into Yoga quite fully, and many schools are available for practice and study under excellent guidance.

The mention of the word Yoga quite frequently conjures up in the minds of many people a picture of rather weird contortionist poses and postures, standing on the head, limbs and spine twisted into all sorts of weird and acrobatic angles, or of an aesthetic-looking person meditating and oblivious to all around. Whilst many of these poses are done, and meditation most certainly practised, Yoga is much more, and has much more to offer.

The importance of breathing in the practice of Yoga, particularly the Hatha Yoga, can be appreciated from the very word 'Hatha', which means sun and moon. The actual interpretation of breathing is that the flow of breath through the right nostril is influenced by the sun, and that through the left nostril by the moon. The word Yoga itself is meant to be a joining of the breaths, and also a joining or realization and union with the Universal Being. This important basis of Yoga is illustrated in a special single nostril breathing exercise.

The wisdom of evolving a system which aims, as Yoga does, at prolonging the physical vigour and life span, can be realized when one appreciates the fact that we rarely reach a stage of wisdom until our bodies are so old that the physical health and vigour are decreasing and degenerating.

The question naturally arises as to how Yoga can achieve this youth and health prolonging effect; how does it work, and what does it do precisely? What does it rejuvenate, and how does it extend the procreative functions and life giving vitality. The breath control and the tonic effect of deep and vital breathing is a powerful agent in purification of the body. So much ageing is due to toxic accumulation, the clogging of the body with waste products, that vital function is greatly lessened. The Asanas or exercise poses affect the whole body. There is an Asana for every organ, every muscle, every joint, and in fact for every single part of the body, and every endocrine gland and glands of external and duct secretion. The flow of nerve energy stimulated to every gland, organ, nerve and muscle of the body, plus the increased blood flow, is the prime factor in the greatly improved functioning of the body as a whole.

Yoga does not make any specific claims for being a panacea or cure-all for disease, but serves more as a preventative and preserver of youthful health, but nevertheless I have seen many diseases and chronic conditions completely and permanently cured after regular conscientious Yoga practice. After all, strengthening the vital organic functioning of the body, together with increased efficiency of the digestive system, and with better gland functions, including the gonads, must have delaying effects on ageing and wear and tear. The importance of healthful functioning of the endocrine glands in the health of the body, physical and mental, is all too clearly seen and appreciated when one or more of these vital glandular functions begins to slow down. Witness the sluggishness, mental and physical, in the middle and old age person, whose thyroid is losing its efficiency and hormone; the lack of vigour and youthful pep when the sex glands are failing; the overall physical and mental slowing up when these vital secretions into our blood stream are lessening. Yoga increases the vital blood flow to and through all the endocrine glands, with natural tonic and stimulating results.

Age is no bar to the commencing of Yoga. Moderation of the more difficult poses is, of course, advised for old people, and some poses must not be done at all. There are also contra-indications in many cases, and thorough medical checks are advisable, but the general practice of Yoga is really open for any age for beginner.

There is no need to change your religion, become a vegetarian, or a celibate, for the average Hatha Yoga student. We have to use and adapt Yoga to a certain degree to fit in with our Western way of life and standards, and common sense must prevail. We do not have the practical need, nor indeed the practical use, for the advanced and higher forms of spiritual achievement reached by the aesthetics of the East. The average person, particularly the average woman taking up Yoga, does so to improve her looks, her personality and magnetism, her health, and to prolong youth.

One of the effects of Yoga Asanas is the restoration, or more strictly the counter effect of the pull of gravity on the organs and tissues of the body. This is accomplished by the inverted poses—the headstand, the shoulder stand, and the half shoulder stand. Many other poses also bring in these effects, particularly uddiyana bandha or stomach lifts, and certain breathing techniques. The flushing of circulation with pressure through certain areas is a feature of some of the poses, and the stretching of the spinal column produces freedom and flexibility plus an increased circulation to the vital autonomic nervous system, as well as the spinal cord itself.

When practising Yoga Asanas and breathing, one must keep in mind that the purpose of Yoga is health, harmonious functioning of the glands, nerves and organs, and not for the gain of big muscles. Large muscles do not necessarily mean perfect health. The Yoga philosophy teaches that the purification and healthful functioning of the body is an indispensable step for the attainment of the mental serenity and realization and union with the universal spirit.

Yoga teaches one to harness the vital life force, instead of dissipating it; it will teach you how to relax, how to master anger, frustration, impatience, hate, passion, greed, and many other harmful emotions which so take hold of us. It will teach how to concentrate on the forces of love and beauty and goodness, it will strengthen the will and the power to focus the mind on the happy, important and health promoting forces within you. The Asanas and the breathing will calm the anxiety, bring a serene outlook. Compulsive eating will be conquered. Although Yoga is not specifically a reducing system, it nevertheless frequently results in loss of excess weight, because of the peace of mind, and elimination of the frustration, dissatisfaction, unhappiness and worrying tensions which so often lead to the over-indulgence or over-compensation with food. At the opposite end of the weight picture, we have the thin, scraggy underweight body benefiting from the improved digestive capacity, because of a calmer and happier frame of mind. This results in a greatly improved assimilation of the food eaten, with resultant weight gain.

Amongst the benefits that Yoga Asanas can bring is the very important one of improving the sex function in women as well as men. Certain Asanas improve circulation and nerve force to the reproductive organs, resulting in a prolonging of the manufacture of sex hormones, and a delaying of the menopause. This factor itself is most important in the retention of youthful looks and vitality. When menopause finally comes, it is entered into and passed through almost unnoticed and without the physical and mental difficulties and disturbances that women have come to expect and fear. Sex life need not be finished, and this certainly could be a factor in the ego and mental outlook of feeling young. For women who suffer sexual weakness or debility, Yoga offers considerable help in the improvement of healthful desire with the confidence and mental content of feeling that they are normal and female. Lack of sex desire or drive should not be confused with or mistaken for sexual frigidity, which is a different thing and is almost always psychological in origin.

The practice of Yoga Asanas, such as the inverted group and the Eagle pose and many others, has so often resulted in the elimination of sterility that the Eagle pose in particular has been referred to as the fertility pose, and many a pregnancy has been facetiously blamed on Yoga. Joke as it may be, the fact remains that many cases of sterility have been benefited, and pregnancy follow. The direct pressure of blood flow to the ovaries and through the reproductive system, especially by poses such as the Eagle, plus the increased flow through the thyroid and pituitary glands of the Inversions, undoubtedly brings about the improved functioning that results. The increased flexibility and healthful stretch also results in elimination of congestion and constriction, and the menstrual flow is accompanied by none of the pains and cramps and flushing that so many women have with each period. The strengthening and toning up of the tissues and muscles in the female sex organs by Yoga Asanas results in a firming, and in the retention of, the elasticity which is lost after childbirth, and which can bring on so many disorders.

Pre-natal and post-natal exercises as practised are basically akin to Yoga Asanas and breathing, and the woman who practices her Yoga Asanas and specific breathing exercises can expect to have a free and easy birth and speedy restoration to normal activity. An important factor here also is the confidence and calmness of the mental approach to the job of giving birth, and it is in this respect that Yoga can perhaps be superior to the normal pre-natal routines. Certain Asanas must be discontinued as the pregnancy progresses, and any pregnant woman doing Yoga should do so under the guidance of an experienced teacher, and not in her own home on a do-it-yourself basis. Likewise other Asanas must not be attempted if certain diseases are manifest; blood pressure, kidney trouble, diabetes, to name a few. Any woman suffering from such troubles, pregnant or not, should do Yoga under supervision, and with constant medical check-ups. Often the careful selection and practice of some specific Asanas results in great improvement in many such disorders, particularly those that may be of a psychosomatic origin.

For the woman—or man—who for some reason cannot lead a normal sex life, Yoga offers the best and most helpful and healthful avenues of sublimation, and the means by which the person can develop the mental frame of mind to sublimate. Sublimation can be quite healthful, as it is merely the transference or transmuting or channelling of one vital force in another direction where it can be used for purposes of constructive value to the body and mind. The alternative state to sublimation is repression and frustration, with their consequence of neurosis and disordered personality traits, mental ill health, and frequenty physical disorders which are quite basically a psychosomatic manifestation of repressed sexual desire. The practice of Yoga is of tremendous benefit to such cases, and no better advice can be given than that of taking up Yoga.

Yoga teaches one to appreciate the beauty of nature and to look for beauty around one, for that is surely where it is. If we will only stop and look for it, we will find it. If we think beauty, have a happy mind, we will surely see it around us, because we have learnt to seek and see it in everything that Nature displays. Yoga meditation and mental concentration on an object of beauty for the sheer joy and peaceful serenity of the contemplation of beauty is one of the most relaxing of the Yoga teachings, and could be practised with reward by anybody—Yoga devotee or not.

The Hatha Yoga Asanas that will be described here are basic and fairly comprehensive. They will work on the entire body, spinal column, muscles, glands and internal organs. Advanced poses are not necessary for the average woman seeking health, beauty, and the delaying of age. The breathing will cover all the principles of Yoga requirements, and will greatly enlarge the vital capacity of the lungs in addition to the systemic and physiological benefits obtained.

The Asanas should be done on an empty stomach and an empty bowel. Early morning is suitable, but most people prefer evening or late afternoon before the evening meal. It matters not, really; just so long as no food is in the stomach and digesting completed. This can mean 3–4 hours at least after a meal, depending on the type of meal. A light meal is most preferable, no animal fats or heavy meats, fruit or salad being the ideal. Wear loose clothing, be warm, and use a mat—preferably thick for comfort.

Asanas

The sitting poses will not be dealt with here, as the most important of the poses for the requirements of the woman seeking health, beauty and youthfulness, will take up sufficient time. The sitting poses are mostly used for meditation, and should be sufficient to mention here· that lotus position and crosslegged poses can be used for some of the breathing exercises, or the simpler kneeling poses if preferred.

Before commencing the Asanas it will be desirable to limber up. Commence by standing with feet slightly apart, body bent forward and arms hanging loosely down in front, hands almost to floor; sway body across to one side, up and back and around and down to other side. Do 3 circles in each direction. Do a few squats with heels flat, a few neck exercises, and a few arm-swinging movements—20–30 as in back-stroke swimming.

The head stand, or Sirshasan, will not be used, and it is

not advised for the beginner, and certainly not without the supervision of a qualified teacher and Yoga expert. There are too many contra-indications, too many difficulties, and it is a controversial matter even among Yoga teachers and experts. It is, however, an excellent pose, but needs expert guidance and supervision.

(1) *Sarvangasan*—shoulder stand—a candle pose

An inversion pose which benefits the whole body, particularly the thyroid gland with increased blood supply, and which in turn influences the whole body. Fig. 17.

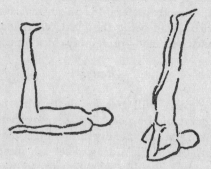

FIG. 17. Sarvangasan (shoulder stand)
Stage One (left) Two (right)

Lie flat on floor, raise the legs, lift the hips and body until quite vertical in one straight line resting on the back of the neck and shoulders only, chin tightly locked into chest; elbows resting on ground and hands pressed firmly into back. *Breathe slowly* and *deeply*, using an *outward bulge* of the *abdomen* with inspiration and contracting abdomen inward on expiration. Hold in beginning for 30 seconds and increase to 3 minutes. Lower gently.

(2) *Matsyasan*—or fish pose

Lie flat on floor, arch back and rest on top of head, with neck well bent and head well under, shoulders off the floor. Arms are by the side, resting on elbows. A more advanced variation is to bring the knees up and cross the ankles. Breathe deeply and slowly and hold for 30 seconds –2 minutes. Fig. 18.

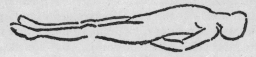

FIG. 18. Matsyasan (fish)

Benefits. The stretching of the front of the neck after the compression of the neck from the shoulder stand brings about a greatly increased blood flow through the neck and thyroid, hence the benefit to this vital gland and the brain.

(3) *Halasan*—the plough pose

So called because it resembles a plough when in completed position. Fig. 19.

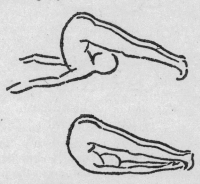

FIG. 19. Halasan (plough) Variation (below)

Lie on back, keep hands, palms down, beside the thighs; keeping legs straight, slowly bring them up and over the head, toes touching the floor; knees must be straight; press chin to chest, breathe slowly through the nose; hold pose for 2 minutes if able, then slowly raise legs and bring back to floor, lying flat on back. Repeat 2–3 times.

Benefits. An excellent stretch for the whole spinal column and back muscles, and an excellent retraction for the abdominal area. All the spinal nerves are stimulated, and circulation greatly improved; lumbago and kindred back ailments, also neck aches, fibrositis, etc., are all greatly benefited and eventually disappear.

(4) *Paschimottanasan*—head to knee pose

Lie on back, slowly raise the body, keeping legs straight on floor; exhaling, bend the body forward and take hold of the feet, burying head into knees; hold for 5 seconds–2 minutes; raise the body and resume the supine position. Repeat 3–4 times. Fig. 20.

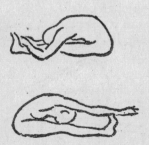

FIG. 20. Paschimottanasan
Variation (below)

Benefits. An excellent abdominal exercise; stimulates liver, bowel, and all the viscera, stretches the hamstrings at the back of the thigh, tones up the spinal nerves.

(5) *Bhujangasan.* Cobra pose

Named because when extended in full position it resembles the cobra snake. Fig. 21.

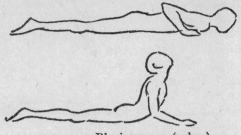

FIG. 21. Bhujangasan (cobra)
Stage One (above)   Two (below)

Lie on floor, face downwards; place hands, palms down, on the floor under the shoulders. Raise head and upper body as a cobra would raise its hood, bending the back well back slowly and a few inches at a time, but do *not* allow the *lower* body to leave the floor—from the navel down the body must be firmly on the floor. Hold for $\frac{1}{2}$–$1\frac{1}{2}$ minutes and lower slowly. Repeat 3–6 times as desired.

Benefits. One of the best exercises for keeping the spine elastic; an excellent toning for all the deep muscles of the back, and a very fine tonic for sluggish bowel and poor circulation through the viscera.

(6) *Salabhasan*—or locust pose

Gives appearance of locust with tail raised when pose demonstrated. Fig. 22.

Lie face downwards, hands alongside thighs, palms uppermost; inhale slowly; keep face on floor, tense back muscles, and lift legs straight and stiff off the floor, also endeavour to lift pelvis as high as possible, press backs of hands firmly into floor, keep the back as arched as possible. Hold for

20–30 seconds; exhale slowly and lower legs down slowly. Repeat 3–4 times.

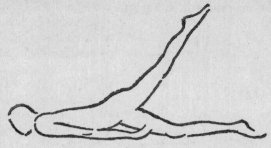

FIG. 22.   Salabhasan (locust)

Benefits. Salabhasan locust pose exercises the lower lumbar and sacral regions of the back, tones the liver, pancreas and kidneys, improves flexibility of lumbar and sacral regions and circulation throughout. The Humbhak, or breath retention during the pose, strengthens the lung and breathing.

(7) *Dhanurasan*—a bow pose

This represents the bow appearance of string and wood of a bow. Fig. 23.

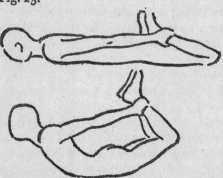

FIG. 23.   Dhanurasan   Stage One (above)   Two (below)

Lie face downward—prone on floor. Bend legs back and grasp ankles. Raise head, body and legs as high as possible to make a bow, using legs to pull arms and body up high; hold for a few seconds (10–30) and lower. Do not jerk up or down, be steady. You may breathe normally or retain breath while up in bow, depending on condition and progress. Repeat 3–4 times.

Benefits. Combines the benefits of Bhajangasan and Salabhasan. These three poses form one complete set for the whole of the spine, and complete an excellent combination of benefits for the vertebrae, nerves and muscles, as well as being an excellent tonic for the liver, kidneys and internal organs generally.

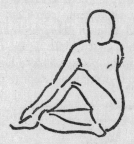

FIG. 24   Ardha-Matsyendrasan
(spinal twist)

(8) *Ardha—Matsyendrasan*—or Spinal Twist

Sit on floor, legs stretched out; bend right leg up and place foot against the perineum or near the groin; bring up left foot and place over the bent right knee, and rest it on the floor outside the right thigh. Pass the right hand and arm around the outside of the left knee, and take hold of the left foot under the instep. The left knee will now be under the right axilla. Place left arm behind back as far round as you can, grasping thigh or clothing for leverage;

turn head over left shoulder, chin tucked in, sit tall and twist body to left. Hold for 5–30 seconds and release slowly. Repeat twist on other side, reversing the leg and arm positions. Repeat twice each side. You can increase the time of holding the pose as you improve. Fig. 24.

Benefits. Keeps the spine elastic and benefits the spinal nerve roots, increases blood supply to the ligaments and deep muscles; good for constipation, dyspepsia, lumbago and rheumatic back troubles. An excellent all round nerve and ligament benefit, improves posture and induces graceful carriage.

(9) *Trikonasan*—Triangle pose

Stand erect with feet about 2 feet 6 inches apart, arms out sideways from shoulders, palms downwards. Bend to left until left hand touches floor, right arm being straight out parallel to floor to the left. Hold for 5–20 seconds, return slowly to upright and bend to right side and hold 5–20 seconds; keep legs straight. Repeat 3–4 times. Fig. 25.

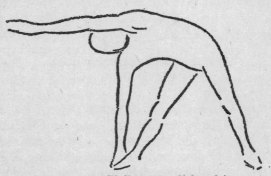

FIG. 25. Trikonasan (triangle)

Benefits. Tonic for spinal nerves and abdominal organs, and bowels. Improves lateral flexibility of spine, and muscles on both sides.

(10) *Savasan*—dead body pose

This is the premier relaxation pose. It should be done at the end of your Yoga session for 5–10 minutes. It can also be done for 30 seconds to 1 minute between each pose. For relaxation between poses, done when lying prone, or face down, such as cobra, locust and bow, position of feet will be slightly altered as explained further on. Fig. 26.

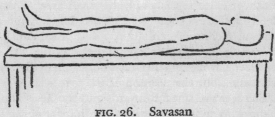

FIG. 26. Savasan

Technique of Savasan: Lie flat on floor in supine position —on back, hands on floor beside thighs, heels together, toes rolled outwards. Begin thinking (eyes closed) of relaxing the feet, allowing all parts of the feet to flop and feel loose and limp, breathe slowly, keep the mind free from all thoughts other than this feeling of loose, limp and sagging relaxation, like a rag doll. Proceed up the body little by little, with this letting go and sagging of each part —the legs, thighs, stomach, etc.; think of all the organs just relaxing, being limp and loose; allow the jaw to sag, do not close mouth tightly, let the neck muscles and face feel loose and heavy and expressionless. Think of peace, serenity, ease, comfort, beauty, and allow no other thoughts to take hold of consciousness; be aware only of your body sagging away beneath you, and your mind floating free of care and tension. You must keep your mind feeling and thinking thus, and the whole body must feel limp, loose and sagging, with the mind light, happy and peaceful.

The benefits of this Savasan pose are temendous. It can be done any time when tension, fatigue and stress are prevalent, and if practised regularly can produce benefits and feelings that are not found with any other poses, but it must be done with complete mental control of letting go and not allowing thoughts to take hold of the mind, because one small thought other than the relaxation technique can produce tension of some small area. This pose completely recharges your nerve vitality battery, and gives a wonderful feeling of exhilaration and peace and happiness. When doing relaxation between poses that are done prone—face downwards—the technique mentally is exactly the same, but the position of the feet is slightly different. The toes are turned inwards and the heels flap outwards, the arms are up across the floor in front of the head, and face resting on the side with jaw sagging loosely.

It will be realized on revision that these poses give a movement for every direction in which the spine can be exercised, flexion, hyper-extension, rotation and lateral flexion. Also that the abdominal organs thoroughly benefited from stretch, squeeze and massage. The lungs and chest also are moved, stretched, and used for utmost benefit.

(11) Uddiyana Bandha

This is a powerful purifying exercise involving a stomach lift. It is a very good stomach, bowel and liver cleanser, an excellent digestion tonic, and is invigorating to the whole system. Done in standing position, as illustrated in Fig. 27.

Empty the lungs by strongly forcing out all of the breath you can; hold breath out draw the stomach up and back as far in towards the spine as you can, hold for about 10 seconds, relax and breathe in. You can also do this with a series of pumping movements whilst holding the breath after expiration. When doing Uddiyana, the hands may be placed on the thighs with body slightly bent forward.

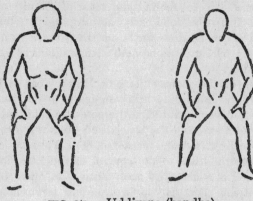

FIG. 27.   Uddiyana (bandha)

Premier breathing exercise—Sukh Purvak

Single nostril breathing exercise with retention.

Sit comfortable with legs crossed or kneeling, body relaxed, mind quiet. Close the right nostril with right thumb, and breathe in deeply and slowly through the left nostril. Then close the left nostril with 4th and 5th fingers of right hand, so that you now have both nostrils closed. Retain for length of time to be decided on, and then lift thumb and exhale slowly through right nostril; next breathe in through right nostril, then close it and hold both nostrils shut, then breathe out through left nostril, after lifting 4th and 5th fingers.

The ratio of inspiration retention (with both nostrils held shut) and expiration (Purak, Kumbaah and Rechak) is 1 : 4 : 2. You can start with 3 seconds inspiration, 12 seconds retention, 6 seconds expiration and increase to 5 : 20 :

10, but whatever time you can do the ratio must still be
1 : 4 : 2. Do 4–6 times.

This breathing exercise purifies the whole respiratory
system and is an excellent relaxant and digestion tonic.
It brings a peaceful feeling and sense of serenity and relaxation. It can be done early morning and last thing on
retiring; it can be done any time when tension and irritability are felt, and can be used with Savasana as a relaxation inducer.

As one of the main objects of Hatha Yoga is breath
control, it is important that you learn to do this. The
breathing movements during the poses, and the retention,
are all necessary, and the specialized breathing described
should be practised and mastered. The Yoga belief that
breath control leads to the control of the Life Force or
Prava itself is a necessary acceptance. You must think of
the purifying effect as you breathe and feel relaxed; do
not strain, but feel the tension flowing out with each
expiration.

It is not possible within the scope of this book to go into
deep pranayama or breath control technique. The breathing described here will provide the benefit for the beginner
in Hatha Yoga. The two most important are the Uddiyana
Bandha and the single nostril inspiration and retention
with expiration in ratio of 1 : 4 : 2.

Simple Breathing Exercises

The following simpler breathing exercises may be used
perhaps in the beginning, or as a preliminary to the others,
and in fact later on included in the full Yoga session of
breathing exercises.

(1) Standing erect, slowly inhale through both hostrils,
retain as long as comfortably able, then exhale right out.

(2) Same as above, but while retaining breath, tense the
whole body.

116

(3) The Ha, or cleansing breath. May be done standing or sitting. Sit with legs comfortably crossed and hands clasped behind back. Inhale deeply through the nostrils, hold a few seconds, then, as bending forward head to floor, exhale and expel the breath with a strong blast through the mouth, making the sound Ha; raise the body again to the upright, breathing in through the nose again, and repeat the process. Do three times, preferably at the finish of a breathing series.

(4) Inhale slowly, retain breath, tap the chest at the top vigorously with both hands 10–20 times, exhale and relax. Do 3–5 times.

(5) Lie on back. Breathe in deeply through the nose for a mental count of 5 seconds; retain for 10 seconds, breathe out through pursed up lips with small opening, for a count of 10 seconds. Do 3–5 times.

During all breathing feel relaxed, form a mental image of the breathing nervous centre—solar plexus, and imagine impurities and tension leaving you.

These breathing exercises will greatly improve the vital capacity of the lungs, strengthen the breathing muscles, the diaphragm, intercostals, and with greater control of breath. The purifying effect on the body physiology will be felt with a more peaceful sense of well being, better relaxation and a sounder sleep, a healthier, rosy glow to the cheeks, and a well oxygenated blood stream.

Whether or not you accept the spiritual, religious and other Yoga theories of the vital forces—Prana, etc., you will realize that the actual practice of the Asanas and the breathing does really bring about an increased feeling of well being and relaxed mental attitude.

You will feel younger, you will stay healthy, and you will know that you are a better person mentally, physically, and emotionally for having done Yoga.

CHAPTER EIGHT

Dancing and
Recreational Exercise

There is probably no older form of exercise than dancing. Way back in man's very primitive beginnings dancing was already a form of expression, an outlet, a recreation from the rigours of maintaining an existence in primitive evolution. All native tribes dance and even at man's evolutionary half ape stage there was probably some form of play or activity which closely resembled dancing and developed along definitive rhythmic beats to become an organized pattern of movement which meant something. Rhythm has a place in man's life, and the rhythm of beat, be it on a drum, log, or any object has an effect on the behaviour of a human body. When culture and development reached the stage of actual music, dancing of course became more extensive and to a definite pattern. Native tribes today have dances for almost every occasion, births, marriages, deaths, fertility rites, ceremonial and religious, puberty, war, battle, victory.

The importance and significance of the place of dancing in the existence of primitive man can be appreciated when one realizes just how widespread it is in all races, tribes and nations. It could be safely said that no race, tribe or peoples would not have dancing as an integral part of their living. In fact, the mythological and religious belief would be an important expression in the dances of native people and would influence the very nature of the dance most powerfully.

One of the physical values of dancing for early man would be the usage of muscle groups in a way that perhaps would not be encountered in their daily fight for existence. Further he would have the stimulation of the rhythmic beat and the feeling of expressing himself and enacting some story or event. These latter enable one to disregard fatigue, and continue for longer periods and since even primitive man may have had the laziness so universally indulged in by all of us, he no doubt received the benefits that we get by pushing ourselves with organized, systematic exercise routines. The frenzy into which some native peoples work themselves because of the significance of the dance, religious, fertility, sexual, is such that the physical effort involved reaches the demands equal to and greater than that to which we are prepared to push ourselves in sport. So it can be seen that dancing can have in many instances a greater health value than many sports. The actual exercise involved and done is quite often greater than most sports other than the very violent ones such as boxing, wrestling, and the like.

Today we have dancing in many forms from the simple to the extremely complex and difficult which can be done only after years of rigorous training as instanced in Ballet. The exercise value in classical ballet is of the very highest and the strength in the bodies of the slim and light ballerinas is quite incredible and unappreciated by the vast majority of people. The male ballet dancer is also deceptively strong, and the leaping power of the trained male ballet dancer is superior to many athletes. The stamina required to dance some leading roles in ballet is equal to many sports and far greater than most people realize.

The years of hard training and physical effort required for ballet dancing lay the foundation for the magnificent constitution and beautiful bodies that we see in the dancers. Many carry on into middle age and retain that youthful figure and vitality. The value and benefit of ballet as an exercise place it high on the list of physical activities from which one can choose for health and fitness. In the person not sufficiently talented, or the person not wishing to make it a career, it is still well nigh one of the best exercises. The beautiful posture, the graceful carriage and movement so characteristic of the trained ballet dancer is something that very few, if any, sports or games can offer or produce. It is to be highly recommended for all posture defects, leg weaknesses and general bodily shortcomings of graceful movement and co-ordination.

National dancing or dancing expressing the very character of a country or race of people is, because of its very nature, widely divergent. The religious beliefs and history involved, do, to a certain degree, minimize the appreciation of national dancing to those of us who do not understand the significance behind it, but we can nevertheless quite appreciate the physical training involved and admire the fitness of the performers.

Whatever exercise one practices or sport that one may play I would advise dancing in some form. The recreational value is tremendous and the exercise an excellent change and variation of bodily muscular co-ordination from physical training routines and games. Ballroom dancing is the most readily available for the majority and is probably more beneficial to the average person than any other form. A greater appreciation of it and far greater exercise value is obtained if it is properly learned and practised. Ballroom studios and schools are within reach of everybody and should be readily used. A far better mental enjoyment is found when one can perform the modern dances and old time dances also with variety and technique; and inferiority feelings are eliminated. The social popularity of a good dancer is well evidenced by the invitations and seeking of such company.

The value of dancing, particularly ballroom for the relief of tension and the cares and worries of everyday living rates the highest. The effect of music, good company, exercise, and the happy atmosphere prevailing all work together in producing the relaxation so needed and sought after. Loneliness is more common than most people realize and what better opportunity to avoid or overcome it than the dance floor with the happy atmosphere of dancing companionship. Many a neurosis has been resolved through dance floor activity.

Whilst dancing is undoubtedly one of the finest of exercises the main reason that the majority of people attend Ballroom dances is because they like it and enjoy the social contacts and happy atmosphere. This in itself is of course a very beneficial factor, the psychological effects of happiness and enjoyment being well known for healthful and relaxing influence. When we add to this mental uplift of what we may call a side effect benefit—the excellent exercise—we have indeed one of the best all round combinations of mental and physiological health and fitness promotion. Whether a person likes exercising or not the fact remains that they are getting it in any case by dancing. There are, however, unfortunately quite a few lazy dancers who merely shuffle around the dance floor and thereby miss out on the benefits of the exercise available to them. These people either cannot dance or merely are interested in the opposite sex and use the ballroom as a medium for contact. They would avoid exercise anyway, so little can be done to induce them to think of health.

The recreational value of pastimes which automatically would bring in exercise such as dancing does, has the added factor in its favour of providing the person who normally would not take to exercise, with such exercise without actually being aware of it. It is well known and realized by all of us just how little we notice the physical exercise accompanying the participation in something of a recreational and socially enjoyable nature like dancing. This factor is one which makes dancing one of the finest, if not the finest, pastime. It is ideal for the person who as they say 'hates exercise'. Add to this the fact that dancing as an exercise rates so highly, we can see the reason and value of including it in our activities whether or not we do any other form of specific exercise for reasons of exercise alone.

Amongst the recreational pastimes which rank similar to dancing where the exercise is perhaps a 'fringe benefit' compared to the principal reason for indulging, we could include some of the social games of activities. Gardening can be perhaps in this category as most people, I think, would attend to their garden for the domestic appearance rather than the exercise.

Swimming to the average person is mostly done for its refreshing and social enjoyment but the exercise performed is one of the best. We must, of course, realize that a large number of people merely dive in and swim only a few strokes at a time but even this is preferable to no exercise at all. Table tennis and indoor games of similar social activities are also beneficial in this respect. Doing something we enjoy in pleasant company, be it competitive or merely a playful pastime is good for us and if that pastime brings in or necessitates physical effort so much the better for us. We should include as many of these activities and pastimes as we can manage in addition to specific and systematic exercise programmes. Golf, tennis, bowls, croquet and the like all have their place in our healthful living programme of keeping fit and keeping young. Those that are done in the open air are preferable and should rate a high priority on our list, but dancing may be the exception because of its greater value mentally and physically.

Amongst recreational outdoor activities it is generally agreed that none could rank higher than hiking through hills and bush. Here perhaps we have a pastime which could be thought of as being done with a higher proportion of reason for indulging, being for the exercise value. It takes more time and as it mostly is just simply walking it would seem that a certain keenness for exercise would be a pre-requisite for partaking. Love of bush and fresh mountain air would influence many in walking but walking for exercise sake gives a person the added incentive to keep going and cover more miles. Like most recreational exercise activities hiking is for both sexes and so has the social company that is necessary for some people to be induced into partaking. Whatever the reasons, attractions, or spurs, the value of hiking through bush and over hills is tremendous and most definitely recommended. Distances covered should be considerable and not merely a slow stroll for a few miles. A minimum of 10 miles is desirable and an all day hike of 20 miles could quite easily be done by most people.

I do not regard motoring as a recreational activity and most definitely do not recommend it, in fact, I would condemn it. In similar category do I include picnics of the type where one drives to a particular spot, sits down and eats, and merely drives home again. It is all too true these latter 'recreations' are so largely indulged in and regarded by too many people as their exercise. Mere sightseeing from a car is a useless physical activity and provides no relief from the strain of driving and further would keep one in the atmosphere of the polluted air of the roadways. We must get out and walk, run or play, breathe, puff and laugh, do something other than sit.

A side effect or fringe benefit of being able to dance can be seen in the business, social functions such as dinners, cabarets and such. These business social activities are much more relaxing and less tension producing if people are able to dance well. The inferiority feelings of being out of such activities through inability to dance are not to a person's advantage but the ability to dance well and combine business with pleasure and entertain has a happier influence on the personality reaction and the popularity rating also. Since wives can often have considerable influence on a business man's decisions the dancing ability and social rating of a business client could improve his status.

The ability to mix with all age groups can have a decided influence on keeping a person's thoughts youthful. No matter what age he be, a good dancer is welcome in any age group and the influence and effect of young people's company on the ego and morale of an older person is indeed quite extensive and beneficial. To be young, look young, and act young as well as feel young, we can use to good advantage the society of young people, and to have them accept our company we must be able to do the things they do. What better start than to be able to dance and keep up with them. It would be advisable, or should I say necessary to learn the new dance crazes as they come into fashion, and since these are not really strict dance steps it presents no problem technically, but is merely a physical fitness requisite.

Recreational activities which entail a rather vigorous physical effort are not as readily indulged in as the lighter variety. Man's inherent laziness would instinctively lead him to easier activities unless some thought on the matter awakens him to the need for more vigorous action. We. must not fall for the 'too old' excuse; vigorous activity is possible to a ripe old age if fitness is maintained. We must do the more vigorous things more often, dance with energy, hike with pep and bounce, do not slacken when we reach a hill. At the same time we must avoid at all costs any nervous haste, remember the objective is recreational activity and exercise, not competitive tension.

For better health and to maintain a youthful, mental outlook some form of recreational activity or activities is essential to augment the more specific health routine of special exercise or yoga. We need variety and we need to enjoy it. Life is for living and to live it to the utmost we need the best health we can get. No time to waste being sick and tired; be healthy and stay younger.

One of the most popular of recreational exercise activities is golf. Apart from the big business of professional tournaments and the competition of amateur tournaments, golf for the average person, be he a business or professional man, is a welcome break from the office desk and provides healthful outing in parkland surroundings with plenty of walking. Golf itself, the action of hitting the ball, is not really of any great value as an exercise other than a good twisting movement for the waist line and as the number of hits is not that many, the main value of golf would appear to be the walking and mental recreation.

The keenness of some golfers, however, is such that the recreational angle tends to be overrun. If the poor scores and bad hits tend to produce irritability, with rising tension, and perhaps a slight elevation of the blood pressure, then that type of player with that type of temperament should reconsider the value of golf as a recreational relaxant. The objective should be to bring about relaxation, not rising temper and tension. We should use certain pastimes for what they are—recreational relaxants and thereby obtain what benefits are available.

Although pastimes of a relaxing nature without too keen a competitive angle should be undertaken with the idea of getting healthful relaxation, we should not go to the extreme and play so lazily that there remains very little exercise in it. We should make it quite an energetic play but keep the mental side distinct from the tense and burning determination to win at all costs. We should strive to win, of course, but should not be intensely anxious to the extent of defeating the very purpose of the game, viz. relaxation and health.

For the person, however, whose ability is tops the game can of course be worth some mental and physical taxing and this person may need then to depend on some other pastimes as a recreation and relaxant. After all if a person is good enough to be top class and win then by all means win and strive to do so but make sure that fitness is behind you to enable you to stand up to the wear and tear. I think it is good health practice to have games or sport we wish to play hard and excel in, with competitive training, and others to participate in for the healthful relaxation and with less serious frame of mind. Balance is desirable and healthful.

Recreational activities or pastimes which do not involve some movement or exercise must be given a minor priority and are best reserved for times when other more healthful activity has been indulged in and rest is called for. In this category we would include card playing, reading, etc. Mental exercise such as the latter is needed as a balance to physical exercise. We need a sharp wit as well as a tuned body.

Mere reading of novels, articles, etc., is not really enough. We should be actually studying and learning something continually. The capacity of the human brain is virtually unlimited and we can literally go on learning until the day we die. Striving to improve mentally as well as physically is necessary for a balanced and healthful existence. Our mind needs to be cultivated as well as our body and we should feed it, exercise it, give it something to chew over, digest and assimilate. Idleness is detrimental, we should avoid it, mentally as well as physically and balance our daily activity for the maximum benefit of our person, as a whole in our striving to stay healthy and keep young.

No recreational activity listings would be complete without at least a passing mention of one very commonly indulged in—drinking. Many people would insist that drinking be considered a recreation. I do not agree; it can be an escape from facing up to tensions and worries of every day living but is definitely not a recreational, healthful balance for such tension. I do agree however, that a social drink is of value as a relaxant but excesses and regular reliance on alcohol can lead to only one unhealthful end—alcoholism. Even moderately heavy drinking brings about degeneration in some degree mentally, and the physical effects such as potbelly and liver cirrhosis are well known.

The value of music, be it listening or playing some instrument, is probably not fully realized as a relaxing medium. Listening to music that one can enjoy, after a session of physical exercise is an ideal balance and healthful relaxant. We can all of us, appreciate beautiful music and should make it a part of our lives. Balance is vital in a health programme, we must have exercise, recreation, fun games, music, seek happiness, for in the harmonious balance of these we have the ingredients to be healthy and stay young.

CHAPTER NINE

Specific and Remedial Health Routines

The animal body has within itself remarkable powers of self healing and curative properties. Too often we hinder this process of natural cure by ignorant interference with nature. Symptom suppression with excessive use of pain killers and germ killers whilst leaving the basic underlying cause untreated can so often leave the disorder merely in a state of chronic quiescence ever ready to flare up again. The body's natural resistance and ability to cleanse itself is hindered, and no real 'cure' may be achieved. For complete cure of any disease the fundamental underlying condition which permits disease to flourish must be removed. It is an unfortunate fact that too often this basic cause is not recognized and accepted. In any case it is far easier to treat a symptom. The fact that some disorders do tend to clear up is a tribute to the power of nature to heal despite interference and hindrance. We should have faith in nature and the body's own wonderful healing power.

Undoubtedly one of the most common causes of many of man's ills is the food he eats, and the excessive amounts of it. In fact, when the tremendous damage of cigarette smoking is considered, we might say that a large percentage of man's health problems is caused by what passes between his lips. Excessive eating, insufficient exercise, polluted air, mental tension, all combine to play their part in bringing about the ill health and poorly functioning condition of the body. Adding insult to injury by treating fatigue with pep pills, highly strung tension with sedatives, vitamin and mineral deficiencies with tonics, can only result in depleting the body of its own vitality still further.

A lamentable shortcoming in the make-up of human nature is the habit of short cut or easy way of treating some disorder. Anything that will permit them to continue eating the food they like—usually a devitalized, denatured or over-sugared one is sought after by some people as a treatment. Symptom awareness with basic causes unrecognized is all too common, and the treatment of symptoms is the only line of action; people will not change this way of living to a healthful pattern which would eliminate the underlying conditions conducive to disease and poorly functioning physiologies. A body clogged with waste and toxic accumulation, constipated, catarrhal and congested is using up a large portion of its vital force in attempting to cleanse itself and rid itself of these fatigue producing conditions. The body is self purifying and will always tend to cleanse itself and keep the blood stream pure and endeavour to fight, neutralize and eliminate poisons, toxic wastes and foreign materials. This is greatly helped by exercise; but the lack of exercise plus the regular eating of excessive food is a constant hindrance, and gives the body very little chance to catch up on this process of self purification. It is only when we 'get sick' and cannot eat, and have a few days of high temperature that we can burn up and catch up.

As pointed out earlier, the value of fasting to the body is little appreciated by the average person today. Even a 24–36 hour fast every few weeks can do a great deal in keeping the body at top tuning in the battle to keep clean internally and be healthy. The habit of fruit only for one day per week is one well worth cultivating also. A three day fast once or twice a year is no hardship and should be undertaken by all of us. Most people would gain more health benefit from such a regime than the annual holiday which more often than not consists of overeating and under sleeping. Many health experts indulge in fasts at 3, 7, or 10 days once or twice a year and this is more of a holiday than any trip away, because it gives the body what it really needs—a rest from overeating, and a chance to lower the toxic accumulation level.

The suggestion that they refrain from eating for even one day causes almost panic state in some people. The old idea that one must eat to keep up one's strength is so ground into man's thinking that fear becomes the main obstacle to even a short fast. We can go many days without food before we actually lose muscle power. It is inconceivable that Mother Nature did not, throughout the process of evolution, provide the body with the ability to tide over periods of food shortage. Ample reserve of vitality is evident.

The liver and the fat storage all provide reserves of potential energy to maintain us. As most people of today carry so much more excess weight than primitive man probably carried, fasting for one day or so should present no real hardship.

The practice of healthful living with proper diet, plenty of exercise, right mental attitude and relaxation in most cases will do much to prevent any condition existing which allows disease to catch on. Resistance to infection cannot be built on poor material; vitamin and mineral deficient food provides or contributes nothing to maintaining high resistance. The unclean condition of the alimentary tract further adds to the burden of the body in its fight for health. Sluggish liver function is very common and is very largely responsible for the chronic fatigue so prevalent. Overeating probably causes more afternoon drowsiness than most other practices, and a heavy lunch is one bad habit we could do without. The specific treatment via exercise and diet of many common disorders is aimed at the basic or fundamental condition of the body which permits lowered resistance of fatigue, disease, and the stresses of modern living. It cannot be accomplished in a few days or even weeks; there is no quick cure like the drug treatment of symptoms or germs, no wonder quick relief; but there will be no side effects, harmful or mild to plague the body. A very alarming percentage of illness is now being treated, caused by the side effects of drug treatment originally.

The necessity for a health building pattern of living based on regular exercise, low fat diet and relaxation is very well shown in the post coronary treatments and the preventive advice. High on the list of causes of heart attacks are smoking, lack of exercise, high fat diet and nervous tension, all of which would be non-existent in a natural health plan or pattern of physical culture living. Why wait for the first coronary, prevent it now. The very same preventative treatment would also tend to eliminate the causes of many other disorders. Prevention is much easier and more pleasant than curing. Why suffer the pain, loss of time, and the financial burden of getting sick?

Your Heart

If you are a potential heart victim, in other words if you smoke heavily, do no exercise, live on a diet rich in animal fats, refined starch and white sugar products, and have a stress job, here is how you can do something to help prevent it: you should run (less at first) 2–3 miles daily or at least 5 times per week, quit smoking entirely, live on a diet composed largely of fruit, salad vegetables, lean meat, no animal fats but vegetable oils and soya beans, you should eliminate white bread, common salt and white sugar entirely from your diet, and ensure that your diet is rich in lecithin and Vitamin E. If necessary, take natural Vitamin E tablets and lecithin meal products. Remember that animal fats include butter, eggs, cheese, milk and dairy products. To reduce your stress level do yoga daily, particularly the breathing and relaxation poses. It is probably wiser to be on the safe side and also eliminate all starchy foods, even wholemeal bread, but cereals, unpolished or brown rice may be allowed as the one exception, but you must learn to have it without sugar or cow's full cream milk. Soya bean milk or skim powder milk with either honey or molasses is best. You need not completely eliminate alcohol, but be strictly moderate. The diet must be sparing in quantity, but high in mineral, vitamin and adequate in protein. Your weight must be strictly on the light side. Have regular cardiographs and check-ups. Do not fear that exercise will damage your heart. Heavy eating and nervous stress will damage it more if you do no exercise, and if you smoke heavily. As a variation from straight out warming or jogging, you can do alternate walk and jog sessions up to 6 and 7 miles or more. With this type of routine you walk one mile or so, jog one or more, walk one or two, and so on. Any alternation you prefer, but cover at least 5 miles, and as much more as you feel able, with alternative walk, trot, walk, trot, etc. Some days you could even do all walking—but it would need to be 7 or 8 miles. You can even walk one day, run the next, and alternate your walk and run programme that way.

Asthma

One of the most distressing of ailments that affects men, women and children alike is undoubtedly asthma. It is much more common than most people realize and can range from the very mild unnoticed, untreated, no distress type to the very debilitating, distressing and incapacitating degree of making life a misery. Causes can range through allergies, dietetic, catarrhal, psychosomatic and emotional. Children can be sufferers but if some treatment is begun early, cure can be effected so that they reach adulthood relatively free of attacks.

Regardless of whether the attacks be triggered by emotional or allergic causes all asthma victims need to be on a diet of non-mucus forming foods to eliminate the catarrhal congestion and make breathing exercises more effective. First and foremost, there must be the avoidance of dairy products such as pasteurized cow's milk, butter, cheese, eggs, cream. Fried foods, roasts should also be eliminated. Meats must be very lean and well grilled. Common salt, white sugar and white sugar products, white flour and white flour products are taboo, and any starchy foods must be very sparingly eaten. Probably the best grain food would be rice, but it must be the unpolished brown, whole grain rice. Soya bean milk should be used but goat's milk may be used in small amounts occasionally. Soya beans should be used as often as possible as a meat substitute. Fresh fruit, salad vegetables are a daily must, all other vegetables should be cooked in waterless cooking utensils if possible, and tea, coffee and soft drinks avoided. Foods which are said to have therapeutic effects on asthma conditions are pineapple, apricots, onions, parsley, mint, lettuce, and raw cabbage.

The exercise programme will consist of specific or special breathing, and the indulgence in some sport that requires constant, steady deep breathing such as swimming—preferably distance, and running—also preferably distance. The breathing exercises that are very beneficial are the yoga, Uddiyana Bandha, the single nostril 1–4–2 ratio of inspiration, retention and expiration, as outlined in the yoga chapter, and the following activities.

Sit comfortably on floor in legs crossed position. Inhale through the nose mentally counting 5, retain breath for count of 10, and exhale through a small opening of the lips as you would for a whistling position, for the count of 10. The opening of the lips must be small enough for you to need to force hard to get the breath *all* out by the mental count of 10. Do this breath 6–10 times. For the finish of the breathing exercises do the H.A. breath in the yoga programme.

If age, weather or circumstance render running or swimming long distances difficult, or impracticable steady walking at a fairly vigorous pace may be substituted, but cover at least 3 miles daily or 5 times per week of about 3 miles. Do the chest exercises, also the back exercises, and full squats.

Uncover any allergies or underlying, emotional causes if possible and as a final measure practise the yoga Savasana relaxation pose daily, and whenever upset.

Constipation

Do all the exercises for the abdominal region in the exercise chapter—sit ups, knee-fold-ups and twists and yoga Uddiyana daily (morning and night). Run, walk, dance and also swim. The following foods and diet programme are are your specific attack on this common complaint.

Avoid all white bread, white flour products and refined cereals, white sugar, milk and milk products other than yoghourt. Eat plentifully of the following fruits in season, first meal in the morning and some on retiring: Apples, dates, figs, grapes, pears, prunes. The following vegetables —onions, pumpkin, celery and carrot. Have honey in place of sugar, and take regularly, 1 large teaspoonful of molasses first thing in the morning—in a cup of hot water if you wish, and again before your evening meal. You may reduce the dose if you find it too vigorous.

This programme for constipation would also be most helpful for the relief of haemorrhoids, particularly the molasses and pumpkin therapy. The addition of regular eating of pumpkin and ripe bananas, plus jacket cooked potatoes further aids the relief.

High blood pressure relief can be obtained by following the heart trouble therapy, but with some caution regarding the severity of the exercises in the beginning. Specific dietetic measures include the plentiful eating of oranges, soya beans, garlic, peaches and apricots. Rutin and Vitamin C tablets are an excellent measure and Natural Vitamin E in moderate doses also. The general diet, specially low salt intake, should otherwise follow that outlined in the heart health programme. Do yoga Savasana, and avoid undue excitement.

The common cold and general upper respiratory catarrhal conditions and sore throat, sinusitis, etc., all have origins so difficult to avoid. Viruses that produce the common cold are so many that vaccine treatment and prevention is not very successful. However, it has been my experience that a dietary habit which avoids all the mucus forming and catarrhal congestion foods, as dairy products in excess, and starchy foods even wholemeal, is the one which gives one the fewest colds, coughs and respiratory ailments. Overheated air-conditioned living plays its part in leaving us soft and poorly resistant to weather, likewise over-clothing ourselves and dodging inclement weather. We should practise a more hardy living and at least get fresh air for sleeping in, even if we are surrounded during the day by so called, air-conditioned atmosphere. To raise resistance to common cold and kindred ailments, I would suggest that you do *not* dodge the rough weather (cold air does *not* give you a cold) go out in it and do some vigorous exercise; avoid dairy products and refined starchy foods, bread and cereals, get plenty of fruit and salad vegetables, especially oranges, pineapple, tomatoes, carrots and raw cabbage. During seasonal difficulties take

Rose Hip tablets and add garlic tablets to your daily diet. Do the yoga breathing and run from 2–3 miles daily. For sore throats pineapple is excellent, and it also is beneficial to bronchial and sinus troubles.

No matter what common ailment is suffered, the adherence to a diet programme as outlined in previous Chapters and the following of a regular and vigorous exercise programme can do more for the prevention of many illnesses than is generally realised. Sickness is largely the result of wrong living, wrong foods and overeating, lack of vigorous exercise, and the generalized pattern of a soft living habit, the all too body reliance on a pill or tablet to correct a minor ache or pain or sickness. Self medication is dangerous, if you are really ill it could be fatal. See your doctor, have regular check-ups but live health, think health, do healthy things, eat natural foods. If you select your diet from raw fruits and vegetables, whole grain foods, and avoid white sugar and excess animal fats, do plenty of healthful exercise, you will rarely, if ever, require medical treatment.

Blood impurity conditions and anaemia all respond favourably to a diet rich in raw fresh fruits, salads and molasses and soya beans. Certain types of anaemia of course require medical diagnosis and treatment and anybody with anaemic condition should at first ascertain the basic cause and type.

Skin Diseases

Although rarely fatal, skin diseases are nevertheless a very aggravating and sometimes distressing complaint; not to mention the embarrassing and disfiguring effect, and its mental side effect. Despite the inherent factor and the child or baby eczema connection, it is most generally agreed that skin troubles are an outward manifestation of inner ill health or biochemical disorder. Sometimes the avoidance of animal fats and the substitution of plenty of vegetable oils in the diet has very beneficial results. The addition of lecithin rich foods such as soya bean and plenty of raw carrots has likewise a very beneficial effect. Vitamin B in all its complexities is an essential and the stringent avoidance of all white sugar and such products is essential. Basic causes must if possible be recognized, such as rashes brought on by any specific food, but generally the avoidance of white sugar and refined cereals and pasteurized cow's milk is the most important step, plus the plentiful supply of vegetable oils in various foods, soya beans, safflower oil, etc., lecithin rich foods and molasses. Drinks of cider vinegar—1 teaspoonful to a cup of water with a little honey are helpful.

Sea water, sun bathing, and regular exposure to air, even cold air, when exercising are all extremely helpful, and Sauna baths or similar sweat producing measures are also quite good except for some disorders which your doctor would contra-indicate.

Liver and Stomach

Most abused, overworked and grossly and habitually insulted of all organs would possibly be the human stomach and the liver. The amazing conglomeration of rubbish which is shovelled into the stomach and the amounts of it, can only make one wonder at the incredible ability of the human constitution to stand abuse. However, it eventually catches up on the shoveller, and the outraged organ makes its protest known in no mild manner. Apart from the immediate and acute results occasionally such as vomiting and when undigested food passes painfully through the intestines to final diarrhoea, the stomach eventually develops ulcers, digestive weakness or some similar chronic shortcomings.

The liver in its turn can also produce much pain through

congestion generally, and from gallstones, which can be extremely and sickeningly painful. Excess of rich high protein, high fat foods such as eggs and roast meats, and the high fat foods as cream and butter eaten excessively with a general over indulgence no doubt constitute the main abuse of the human liver. If to this is added heavy alcohol consumption it is then no wonder the liver protests painfully. First and foremost in the relief of liver congestion and troubles is the abstinence from food for a period of one to three days, depending on the degree of discomfit. Resumption of eating is best commenced with oranges or orange juice, gradually adding fruit and well chewed salad vegetables. Avoid the heavy fat foods, roasts, fried foods and eggs and cream. Specific foods should include, grapefruit, parsley, apples, dandelion and carrots.

A regular, vigorous exercise programme is a must, and over-eating strictly avoided. Do not eat unless really hungry, if a sedentary worker, two meals per day are ample with a fruit only breakfast. Do yoga Uddiyana and all abdominal exercises and swim or run whenever able, make a habit of pre-breakfast run of 1–2 miles followed by fruit breakfast. If a hard worker, breakfast may include dates, a slice or two of wholemeal bread with polyunsaturated margarine and Marmite or honey. Drink dandelion coffee or herb teas and be very moderate with the consumption of alcohol if you must have it at all. Yoghourt is beneficial to the stomach and assists the digestive process, likewise molasses.

Rheumatism, fibrositis, lumbago, and kindred physical pain are today so universally prevalent in varying degrees that hardly a person escapes completely. A great deal is still not known regarding specific causes. Everything from infective agents, diet, dampness and climate has been blamed. Of these, many, I think may be regarded as influencing the susceptibility of the person rather than being a direct, specific cause. Recent research has shown that people in countries predominantly wheat and rye eating have a higher incidence of rheumatic diseases than others, irrespective of nationality or geographic climate. At the other end of the scale, rice eating people tend to have a lower rate of such diseases.

However, regardless of what genetic, racial, geographical or climatic basis exists or prevails, rheumatic disorders are most likely to afflict the unfit and overfed. The accumulation of toxic wastes undoubtedly provides a suitable base for inflammation of muscle fibres and tendons. Vigorous and regular exercise is necessary to prevent this toxic state. A diet deficient in alkalizing minerals further burdens the body in its efforts to deal with excess acid waste. Vitamin C lack is also found to be a factor and most people suffering from rheumatism are found to have insufficient Vitamin C in their diet.

Cold, damp weather finds an increase in the aches and pains of the rheumatic type, but whether this is due solely and specifically to the cold and damp or more to the fact that people tend to eat less fruit and salads in this weather is not certain. I would say that the latter is more likely. Cold and exposure may certainly stiffen a muscle as most people have learnt, but whether mother nature with her marvellous defences and healing capacity meant this to include actual pain and soreness is very doubtful. Surely the body with its long evolutionary adaptations and survival selections would be able to deal with cold and weather changes.

The overall fight to remain free of muscle pain, joint stiffness, tendon inflammation and painful movement generally, would seem to feature, and centre around keeping the body free of toxic material and excessive waste products by means of regular vigorous exercise to a perspiration level and above all to adhere to a diet free of acid forming and devitalized deficient foods.

Most rheumatism sufferers are found to be on a diet of white bread and devitalized cereals, white sugar and allied products, insufficient Vitamin C, B and E and generally lacking in a mineral rich food intake. Tea and coffee drinking are usual and cigarette smoking also. To be free of rheumatic aches and pains I think it is essential to avoid such foods in the diet, and to subsist on a diet composed largely of fresh fruit and salad vegetables. The only cereal advised would be unpolished rice. Molasses, honey and cider vinegar should be a daily inclusion and the best vegetables, fruit, celery, grapefruit, carrot, asparagus, parsley, cucumber and tomatoes. Adjuncts to the diet of alfalfa tablets, Rosehip Vitamin C, and natural Vitamin E are also advised but the overall factor must be a diet rich in natural fruit and salads to 80% and the balance of unpolished rice, molasses, lean meat and cooked vegetables with soya beans as a regular food.

Of all the disorders that ail mankind, none is more common than the 'common cold', none so prevalent, none so easy to get, none so annoying and time wasting. So many ideas still exist as to the cause or causes, that prejudice and ignorance are the main hurdles encountered in the tracking of prevention or lessening of the amount and number of colds contracted. The very naming of this virus infection by calling it a cold is in itself a misnomer as it has been proved by scientific experiment more than once, that cold does not give one a 'cold'. Some scientists have provided evidence to show that cold does not have any significant effect even on the severity or susceptibility to 'catch cold'.

The first step to building the state of health of resistance to this acute catarrhal congestion and infection is to accept the fact that cold does not cause it. Virus contact and acquisition is the direct proven cause. The next step is to realize why it gets us and how and what condition exists in us to allow it to take hold sometimes, and not at other times. The health and tone of the mucous membranes is of prime importance, the capacity of the body to fight infection is likewise. In this regard it would seem that ample Vitamin A and C are important items. However, irrespective of the body's resistance capacity and vitamin intake, undoubtedly any condition of excessive toxic accumulation with congestive catarrhal conditions of the mucous membranes would provide a suitable starting or breeding ground for invasion of virus attacks. Perhaps we might say at this juncture that a person needs a 'cold' or a virus to initiate the acute eliminative process. In other words, if the 'cold' virus gets you then you need a good cleaning out of toxic accumulation, and the mucous membrane of the respiratory tract is a suitable avenue.

The fact that 'colds' would seem to be more prevalent in wintry weather is not an argument against 'cold' not causing colds. In actual fact, 'colds' are quite often found in the tropics, and rarely in below freezing climates in primitive conditions. It is only in the heated, over crowded air-conditioned soft living of civilization that we find such high incidence. The greater consumption of mucous forming foods and heavier eating generally—particularly of fats—is a much more likely foundation for the thriving of conditions suitable to 'catch a cold'. In winter weather, we stay in-doors more, we eat more bread, butter, cream and fatty foods, and bigger dinners generally, we coddle ourselves too much and we do less exercise. Most people gain weight in winter.

In other words perhaps we *create a condition* rather than 'catch a cold'. It is a fact that there is very little catarrhal conditions acute or chronic in a person whose diet is free of foods which are excessively mucous forming. I have seen children go through childhood with no tonsil, adenoid, or ear, nose or throat troubles, and only on rare occasions with a slight drizzle, on a diet which did not include pasteurized cow's milk, white bread or white sugar and in fact was low in dairy products generally. Conversely, I have seen many a child, chronically catarrhal and prone to all such disorders change from such a diet and become greatly improved and practically free from further catarrhal condition. Some of course, are more susceptible than others, and some lack the ability to handle such foods anyway, whilst others have definite allergies. To avoid 'colds' we must first avoid creating the condition that permits a 'cold' to take hold, i.e., we must *not* dodge cold weather, or coddle ourselves, we must *not* lessen our exercise activity and we must *not* consume excessive fats and starchy foods. Plenty of fruit and a daily salad are essential even in the wintry cold weather, and heavy roast meals and fried foods should be avoided. Soya bean milk is the ideal substitute for pasteurized cow's milk and honey the perfect substitute for white sugar. Pure wholemeal bread and unrefined cereals are the only grain food we need use, and vegetables such as potatoes and root vegetables are ideal winter foods. Carrots are extremely rich in minerals and Vitamin A precursor—carotine, and are a daily must. All citrus fruits are important and are a daily necessity.

The exercise programme should include long walks or runs in the fresh cold air and also solid exercise sessions and two or three good solid sweats per week—sauna baths if desired. Plenty of deep breathing exercises (the yoga breathing is particularly beneficial) are most helpful and once or twice weekly dosage of ultra violet or sun lamp helps further the building of resistance and tone. Although the causative virus may be different for the various other diseases which afflict our upper respiratory tract and likewise the germs which attack our deeper respiratory functioning the fact remains that a regime of living that builds our resistance to one, tends to keep us toned to resist all similar respiratory diseases. The condition of clean mucous membrane, a healthy adaptive skin reaction to temperature change, a clean alimentary tract, high vitamin and mineral and green leaf food diet, and the avoidance of animal fat and mucous forming dairy produce foods is the condition that provides us with the best resistance and leaves us with the least need for eliminative processes to rid us of the excessive toxic accumulation.

A really healthy fit body with the high resistance foods nourishing it, the regular exercise and fresh air toughening it, does not have any fear of adverse effects of exposure to cold, wet conditions or weather changes. Even when and where conditions beyond our control such as working conditions of polluted air, or conversely over-heated, air-conditioned smoky offices prevail, we will not have anywhere near the number or severity of so called 'colds' if we adhere to the right diet, right exercise and live right.

Insomnia

One of the camp followers of civilized living and a disorder of human bodily functioning which gives rise to much worry, most of it unnecessary is the common complaint of insomnia. True insomnia is actually quite rare, most people who claim that they cannot sleep a wink are really exaggerating. Disturbed, troubled, spasmodic, sketchy, patchy sleep is the more likely condition. Difficulty in falling asleep is also a problem with many, likewise falling asleep quickly, but only to awaken after a few hours to toss and turn for the rest of the night.

It is a generally agreed upon fact that much of the harm of insomnia is the worrying about it. If the worry of not sleeping can be lessened or eliminated, not only would very little damage be done, but most probably the person would sleep better anyway. It is here that we have one of our best weapons for improving our sleeping—YOGA!

The conscientious practice of yoga Asanas, breathing and relaxation can work wonders with the relaxation and improvement of the quality and depth of sleep. Quantity may vary with different people, but the most important factor is the quality of the sleep. In addition to the yoga, some vigorous outdoor exercise is essential as it is necessary to be healthily tired and not merely nervously fatigued. Long walks, preferably daily are needed, and deep breathing is most helpful. The realization that one actually does sleep much more than one appears to do is very important. Similarly the realization and belief in the physiological and psychological fact that the loss of a little sleep does not do as much harm or make one feel so ragged as the lying awake worrying about it. Recreational activities are necessary, particularly dancing which ranks high on a programme for better sleeping. We must not worry about the lack of sleep, but instead do something positively active to get healthily tired. Most people are more often nervously fatigued, rather than physically tired, and it is in this condition that relaxation is so hard to obtain. The prime necessity here is hard exercise to make one quite physically tired and to relax or reduce the nervous tension. Fatigue has many causes—physical, nervous or mental, nutritional (Vitamin B lack largely, and Vitamin C), boredom and unhappiness and lack of good quality sleep. All of the causes can be removed by regular vigorous exercise, diet improvement, being busy, healthful relaxation and recreation.

CHAPTER TEN

Natural Health and Physical Culture Living

Getting fit, being healthy, staying young depend more than ever today on a pattern of overall healthful living. No single item or aspect such as exercise alone, strict diet, or the avoidance of dissipating habits is, on its own, sufficient to give us the abounding health and vigour that we need and should have. We need to think health, to be aware of what health is, to live a life wherein health is top priority; for without it we have nothing, whatever else we may possess materially.

We do not have to be fanatics, faddists, or cranks, and we should certainly avoid being hypochondriacs or worriers over every little lapse in our condition. We must not allow ourselves to become pill punishers; most of the little things that go wrong with us from time to time will get better of their own accord by virtue of the body's natural powers of self-remedy. We should bear a little pain occasionally—it is most inadvisable to use powerful drugs for minor complaints. We must remove basic causes of disorders, and allow the body to repair and heal itself. We must be patient, and bear with it during the healing and curing process. Prevention is always the prime factor in a health and fitness programme. Prevention is actually easier than curing and we should realize this, although some people would be inclined to say that exercise is no easy way to health. Laziness is, however, a real cause of poor health and we should not seek to always follow the easy placebo of pill-taking, pep-up or sedation. We should face up to some discomforts occasionally, rough it, uncoddle ourselves and when minor sicknesses or disorders afflict us we should give nature a chance to right us and not rush for pain-killers and drugs. Our own resistance is built up by exercising it, not by subduing it with symptom suppressive measures. Nature cure will take a little longer but the final result is better health, better resistance for any future troubles. Fasting for a few days through the acute stages, natural wholesome diet and health measures work wonders. A programme of exercise and general health building measures will ensure future health and vital resistance to fatigue and disease producing conditions.

It has been said that moderation in all things is a good rule to follow. This may be so to a degree but moderation in dissipation and wrong eating cannot be as healthful as avoiding dissipation and wrong foods altogether. Certainly moderation in the sense of balancing our habits is a healthful thing. Our exercise, our eating, our relaxation and recreation should be balanced and moderation here should apply so that each has its time allocation with the avoidance of rush and hasty indulgence in any particular thing. Moderation in eating is more desirable than any other habits, perhaps because overeating can be so wearing and constitutionally damaging organically.

Chronic fatigue needs to be looked into, the causes ascertained and attended to. The causes are largely overeating, with Vitamin B and C deficiency and mineral lack also. Boredom and dissatisfaction, frustration and generally mental tension, lack of exercise and lack of healthful sleep are also causative factors. The general plan for overcoming chronic fatigue is to attend to all these conditions. Do plenty of hard exercise, also yoga, change the diet to a wholesome one of natural foods, as outlined in Chapter

Three, and be busily and happily employed mentally. Avoid tension and worry, use yoga relaxation and breathing and take up a healthful hobby and an enjoyable recreation. A really fit person on a Vitamin B rich diet needs less sleep because the quality is better. One awakens fresher and feeling rested and ready for the day.

Far too many people today care more about their automobile than their own body and give far more careful attention to its maintenance than to their own bodily health and functioning. Many others give more time and attention to their animals, and the diet of prize animals is far more strictly supervised than the person's own nutrition. It is fortunate indeed for us that the body we have is such a wonderful complex machine and so capable of repairing the ravages of abuse and lack of attention. No man made machine can compare, even the most complex computer.

An overall pattern, creed or system for health and fitness must cover all aspects of constructive, health building living. Overeating, smoking, excessive drinking and over-stimulating indulgences and excesses must be avoided in a plan for staying healthy and being younger. Regular exercise is necessary, strong willpower also, but the important factor mentally is to realize and accept the fact that today, real health and youthfulness has to be earned. Modern civilized conditions of living do not permit perfect health and fitness, too many factors are against the maintaining of the natural health we should have. We need to work for health with mind and body.

It is virtually impossible, of course, to avoid all the unhealthful factors in modern living. Cigarette smoke is all around us, polluted air fills our lungs, chemicals, pesticides and other poisons are in our food, our water, and the insistence in creating conditions for the easy life, the soft living, the excess comforts, is an obnoxious factor favouring degeneration of natural health. Stress, tension, and the fast pace of competitive striving have their demands and the price we pay is far too often more than we can afford healthwise. It is vitally important that we do something to at least offset or counter something of the ill-effects of these insidious, wearing down factors. It is not even enough to merely avoid as many of them as we are able to—we must do something more constructive, not only to attempt to repair damage already done but prepare our body as far as possible to stand up to future ravage. It is not enough to just avoid dissipation, we must build health, strength and fitness, and we must condition our way of thinking to that of health and the necessary realization of the priority it deserves. Without this mental attitude we cannot hope to stay healthy and we will most certainly not be younger.

Care will be necessary in the beginning regarding drastic changes, too suddenly, although some people prefer complete cessation of unhealthy habits. With smoking, I am personally in favour of complete cut out. Dietetic changes can be less drastic, but a short fast greatly assists the change over to healthful natural foods. The cleansing effect of the fast wipes the slate clean so to speak, and the body is then ready for a new start on natural untampered vitality foods.

I am not in favour of rigid schedule in one's daily life, although the working hours and pattern of modern civilized living creates obstacles and difficulties in living any other way. However, I think one can avoid having such a tight schedule as rising at 7.1½ a.m. deep breathing, shower, breakfast, etc. and out by 7.31½ or so. If one retires at different hours on different nights then one should expect to awaken at different hours. Lying in bed merely for the sake of lying in after the sleep requirements have been met is not healthful. Time should be allowed for a no rush routine, time to stretch the body in bed before arising (an excellent habit), time for a few exercises and deep breathing—and perhaps a jog or run of 1–2 miles. Breakfast must not be rushed and in any case, only eaten if really hungry.

Whilst on the healthful habits of early morning for starting the day, I must make mention of a rather unhealthful one—the modern alarm clock. Being awakened out of a sleep by an alarm cannot be anything but harmful. If a person needs to be awakened in such a manner then that person is not getting enough sleep and needs to retire earlier. The healthy fit body, functioning correctly and efficiently will take its quota of sleep and awaken naturally. It behoves a person to retire at such time to enable that quota of sleep to terminate naturally before the hour necessary to arise, particularly so as to allow time for some healthful practice of stretchy exercise, deep breathing or a run.

A very healthful practice is a short nap or rest for an hour or so after the lunch break. This of course, is virtually impossible for the majority of people but at least most could get half an hour after the lunch, even a rest or relaxation pose works wonders. A relaxation frame of mind is a very desirable and quite necessary state for the good digestion of the evening meal and no big dinner, or any meal for that matter, should be approached with the worries of the day still active in the mind, with tension still unresolved. It is at this stage where exercise, particularly the yoga relaxation, has one of its greatest effects for the benefit of our health.

An overall pattern of habit for healthful 'stay younger' living must include the wise use of water—internally and externally. Far too little water is drunk as such, it is usually merely the solvent for some other substance, tea, coffee or synthetic fruit cordial. It is not, however, necessary or really healthful to force water into the body in quantities way beyond the thirst satisfying stage except in rather specific disorders and treatments. We should nevertheless drink more than we do. It is an unfortunate fact that water today is not always as pure as it could be. The external use of water is probably overdone almost as much as it is under-done. Too much use of hot water together with lavish use of soap is not really beneficial to the body particularly the skin. Hot, soapy baths should not be a daily necessity for the average person; more benefits are found with cool showers and plenty of vigorous rubbing whilst in the shower with minimum use of soap. The body's natural oil on the skin is washed off by hot soapy water and the acid-alkali balance upset. In many cases, where sensitive skins exist actual rashes appear. It is a fallacy that one cannot get clean by cool showers and no soap. One can get just as clean but it takes longer and a little more effort but the results are a glowing skin, natural oil retained and circulatory toning. The exhilarating effect and feeling with a cold shower following a sauna bath, or hard vigorous exercise to perspiration stage, is well known.

It is not sufficient to be a diet enthusiast or an exercise addict, or a fresh air fiend to maintain health and youth. Too many diet fanatics regard diet as the only necessity and do not do exercise; too many exercise for fitness cranks eat what they like with little knowledge of nutrition and live only a little longer, if any, than others. A balanced pattern of 'stay healthy, live longer' method of living must include regular and plentiful exercise, natural wholesome food and in amounts sufficient only for necessary normality of weight. The pattern must have the backing of the right mental attitude: one must think about health—discipline is needed. The rewards to the person prepared to exercise the body as nature intended and constructed it for such exercise, who feeds it with as natural a diet as procurable, relaxes it as it should be, are greater than anything money can give—radiant health and preservation of youthful looks and vigour—the reward of staying healthy and being younger.

INDEX

A Selection of Cookery Books from Sphere

The 'Cordon Bleu' Series
The following titles fully illustrated in full colour at 90p each

Further Titles on Health & Medicine Include

All Sphere Books are available at your bookshop or newsagent, or can be ordered from the following address: Sphere Books, Cash Sales Department, P.O. Box 11, Falmouth, Cornwall.

Please send cheque or postal order (no currency), and allow 7p per copy to cover the cost of postage and packing in the U.K. or overseas.